DOSAGE CALCULATIONS IN SI UNITS

MAUREEN OSIS, R.N., M.N.

Clinical Nurse Specialist
Southern Alberta Regional Geriatric Centre
  at the Colonel Belcher Hospital
  Calgary;
Adjunct Assistant Professor, Faculty of Nursing
University of Calgary

SECOND EDITION

Illustrated

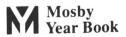 **Mosby
Year Book**

St. Louis   Baltimore   Boston   Chicago   London   Philadelphia   Sydney   Toronto

**Mosby
Year Book**

Dedicated to Publishing Excellence

Editor: Linda Duncan
Project Manager: Peggy Fagen
Book and Cover Design: Gail Morey Hudson
Production: Kathy Teal

SECOND EDITION

Mosby–Year Book, Inc.
11830 Westline Industrial Drive, St. Louis, M

The C.V. Mosby Company Ltd.
5240 Finch Avenue East, Scarborough, Ontario M1S 5A2, Canada

Canadian Cataloging in Publication Data

Osis, M. (Maureen)
    Dosage calculation in SI units

2nd ed.
ISBN 0-8016-3721-X

1. Drugs—Dosage.   2. Pharmaceutical arithmetic.
I. Title.

RS57.O754 1990   615′.14′01513   C90-094594-X

C/B/B   9 8 7 6 5 4 3 2

PREFACE

Over 12 000 Canadian nursing students and practitioners used the first edition of *Dosage Calculations in SI Units*. It was Mosby Ltd.'s first Canadian nursing text, so it is gratifying that it achieved such success. Many of the users evaluated the book and provided helpful information about what to change and what to maintain. This information has been instrumental in the revision.

Features retained from the first edition

Why is the book so successful? Users and reviewers like it because it offers:

- a clear, concise, easy to understand presentation on the skills required for dosage calculation
- the basic concepts for competency in calculations without unnecessary or distracting information
- self-evaluation and self-paced learning through pretests and exercises
- mastery of each concept by requiring 100% on all tests
- the user the opportunity to work through problems on paper as well as solving calculations "intuitively"
- a hierarchical ordering of the modules, moving from the simple to the complex
- Canadian content along with the use of SI units
- an approach appropriate for nursing students faced with the new task of dosage calculation as well as for nursing practitioners who wish to update their skills

These popular features have been retained in the second edition.

New to the second edition

Users and reviewers suggested ways to improve the book. The following changes have been incorporated into the new edition.

SUGGESTIONS

Arithmetic entrance examinations indicate that students have considerable difficulty with decimal numbers.

The first edition provided alternative approaches for dosage calculations: minimal use of rules and formula as well as ratio and proportion. More emphasis is needed on proportion equation as the most versatile and reliable approach. Formula may be forgotten or confused.

Students who have difficulties need more exercises.

REVISIONS

Module 3 is expanded. An appendix for additional practice is added.

The opportunity to master writing and solving proportion equations is increased by 30% through expansion of Module 4 and an appendix. Modules 7 through 10 each present additional examples illustrating calculation with ratio and proportion. For some exercises, the Answer Guide shows the proportion equation, the solution, and the validation of each problem.

The first edition had over 700 questions on arithmetic, conversions, and calculations. This edition has expanded to include over 1 000 questions of which more than one third involve dosage calculations. This represents 50% to 100% more questions than other books of similar page length.

Other features

The book is up to date. Presently, many medications are given by the intravenous route. Errors by this route are significant because the drug is irretrievable. More emphasis is given to both calculation of rate of flow of IV fluids and calculation for reconstitution of medications and infusion via IV fluids.

The approach simulates clinical experience. All dosage calculations are drawn from clinical examples within hospital and community settings. Actual drug labels and syringe diagrams are used.

The book promotes competence through the instructional design and by insisting on 100% mastery.

How to use this book

To the instructor

The book can be used independently or as an adjunct to laboratory or clinical conferences. Module 1 can be used to assess individual students or class performance and identify areas of weakness.

Module 10 is designed specifically for nurses who work in pediatric and critical care settings. This module was expanded in response to many requests from users who said that the book would serve them before and after graduation. If these calculation problems are not needed by your nursing students, simply omit the module or assign only relevant material.

A CAI program is available upon adoption of the book and can be used on Apple or IBM computers.

Appendix E was written with you in mind. Four exams are included — without the answers — for you to use in the clinical area to evaluate students' mathematical and calculation skills before medication administration. You may want to use the multiple choice format for quick marking and computer statistical analysis.

To the student

This book consists of ten modules. Module 1 is a pretest designed to assess your arithmetic and calculation skills. The answers will help you diagnose your strengths and weaknesses. You might want to complete this test before you start the other modules and repeat it after you finish the book.

Modules 2 through 10 each have a pretest, a learning package explaining the specific concepts, exercises to test your understanding, and a posttest. It is recommended that you proceed through the modules in sequence. A further note on Module 10: it is specifically designed for nurses working in pediatric and critical care settings. You will want to complete this module at the appropriate time in your nursing program. You will also want to keep this book; it will serve as a valuable review after graduation.

For each module:

1. Write the pretest to assess your skills.

2. Correct the pretest using the Answer Guide at the end of the text.

3. If you achieve 100% in the pretest, you might choose to omit the module learning package and proceed to the pretest of the next module.

4. If you don't achieve 100% in the pretest, read the module learning package and complete the exercises, concentrating on your weak areas as diagnosed in your pretest score.

5. Correct the exercises using the Answer Guide.

6. Write the posttest at the end of the module without referring to the module learning package or any other resources.

7. Correct the posttest using the Answer Guide.

8. If you achieve 100%, proceed to the next module.

9. If you don't achieve 100% in the posttest, analyze your problems. For example, are your errors related to one skill, such as division of fractions, or are you weak in several skills? Review the appropriate sections of the module's learning package until you improve your skills.

10. Rewrite the posttest.

Note: You are expected to achieve 100% because of the importance of accuracy when calculating drug dosages. You might be tempted to proceed if your test scores are "close" to the mark. However, you are encouraged to diagnose your errors carefully and master the arithmetic or calculation skill before you proceed.

A few students who used *Dosage Calculations in SI Units* in its first edition asked the question: Why do we have to achieve 100% on the tests before moving on to the next module? The answer to that question is another question: would you want to be given IV medications by a nurse who understands only 80% of the task? Surely not, and that is why complete mastery is required.

You will be surprised how your efforts will pay off with 100% accuracy.

Acknowledgment

I want to thank all those who used the first edition and took the time to send both positive evaluation comments and suggestions for improvement. Specifically, I would like to mention Linda Cameron and Alma Funk for their thorough reviews.

In particular, I extend my gratitude to the following individuals who assisted with the second edition: Darlene Aberle, R.N., B.N., Nurse Clinician, and Debbie McNeil, R.N., Clinical Nurse Specialist, NICN, and Harry Morrison for his expertise in arithmetic instruction. I wish to thank Terry Barber of Mosby for his invaluable assistance and encouragement with the second edition. I express my lasting gratitude once again to my family, Imants, Andrew, Lara, and Sean, for their humor, enthusiasm, and support.

Maureen Osis

CONTENTS

Module 1: Arithmetic

PRETEST

Instructions

1. Write the pretest without referring to any resources.

2. Correct the pretest using the answer guide.

3. If your score is 100 percent, you may not need to complete this workbook.

4. If you do not achieve 100 percent accuracy, determine your weak areas and proceed through the workbook.

Arithmetic of Whole Numbers

1. $\begin{array}{r} 546 \\ +677 \end{array}$

2. $\begin{array}{r} 1\ 972 \\ +\ \ 545 \end{array}$

3. $\begin{array}{r} 729 \\ +\ \ 85 \end{array}$

4. $\begin{array}{r} 139 \\ +455 \end{array}$

5. $\begin{array}{r} 831 \\ -\ 356 \end{array}$

6. $\begin{array}{r} 1\ 897 \\ -\ \ 543 \end{array}$

7. $\begin{array}{r} 452 \\ -399 \end{array}$

8. $\begin{array}{r} 894 \\ -\ 105 \end{array}$

9. $\begin{array}{r} 876 \\ \times\ \ 59 \end{array}$

10. $\begin{array}{r} 645 \\ \times\ \ 13 \end{array}$

11. $\begin{array}{r} 3\ 789 \\ \times\ \ \ 235 \end{array}$

12. $\begin{array}{r} 1\ 094 \\ \times 2\ 001 \end{array}$

13. $11\ )\overline{\ 55}$

14. $12\ )\overline{\ 96}$

15. $25\ )\overline{\ 125}$

16. $326\ )\overline{\ 2608}$

YOUR SCORE: _____ %

Note: the Metric Commission of Canada states that spaces are used to separate long numbers into three-digit blocks. With four-digit numbers the space is optional, e.g., 1 972 or 1972; e.g., 123 456.

Arithmetic of Fractions (simplify if necessary)

1. $\dfrac{3}{9} + \dfrac{7}{13} =$

2. $\dfrac{5}{7} + \dfrac{3}{16} =$

3. $\dfrac{1}{6} + \dfrac{3}{5} =$

4. $\dfrac{11}{12} + \dfrac{1}{2} =$

5. $\dfrac{3}{4} - \dfrac{5}{16} =$

6. $\dfrac{11}{12} - \dfrac{2}{3} =$

7. $\dfrac{19}{24} - \dfrac{1}{2} =$

8. $\dfrac{7}{8} - \dfrac{5}{6} =$

9. $4\dfrac{7}{8} \times 5\dfrac{6}{7} =$

10. $2\dfrac{5}{6} \times \dfrac{1}{2} =$

11. $\dfrac{3}{4} \times 9\dfrac{15}{16} =$

12. $3\dfrac{1}{3} \times 2\dfrac{1}{2} =$

13. $\dfrac{7}{8} \div \dfrac{3}{5} =$

14. $\dfrac{9}{16} \div \dfrac{3}{4} =$

15. $3\dfrac{1}{4} \div \dfrac{1}{3} =$

16. $\dfrac{5}{9} \div \dfrac{7}{10} =$

17. Express as a mixed number: $\dfrac{24}{7} =$

18. State the lowest common denominator for $\dfrac{1}{4}$ and $\dfrac{1}{12}$:

19. Express in lowest terms: $\dfrac{18}{72} =$

20. Which of the following is an improper fraction?

　　a. $\dfrac{3}{4}$　　b. $\dfrac{22}{8}$　　c. $1\dfrac{3}{4}$　　d. $\dfrac{1}{10}$

21. Express as an equivalent fraction: $\dfrac{1}{4} = \dfrac{4}{X}$

YOUR SCORE: _____ %

Arithmetic of Decimal Numbers

1. Write "one-half" in correct decimal format.

2. Round to the nearest tenth: 5.67

3. Round to the nearest hundredth: 5.607

4. $2.398 + 5789.78 =$

5. $1\ 298.478 - 983.99 =$

6. $5.67 \times 3.93 =$

7. $3.515 \div 0.95 =$

8. Express this fraction as a decimal number: $\dfrac{7}{8} =$

9. Round the answer to #8 to the nearest tenth.

10. Express this decimal number as a fraction and express in lowest terms: 0.75

11. Arrange in size from largest to smallest: 0.1, 0.01, 0.001, 1.01

Complete the table below to express the ratios as fractions, decimals, and percents. Round decimal numbers to nearest hundredth.

Ratio	Fraction	Decimal	Percent
1:4	12.	13.	14.
5:6	15.	16.	17.
1:1 000	18.	19.	20.

YOUR SCORE: _____ %

Word Problems

1. The first hockey team had ten men on the ice, and six were given penalties for fighting. The second team had seven men on the ice, and all were given penalties for fighting. What percent of players was given penalties?
Answer: _____

2. The parking lot sign states "$0.50 for each quarter hour". You park from 1:17 to 3:35 pm. How much will you pay for parking?
Answer: _____

3. There are ten women in the class, and there are twice as many men as women. How many people are in the class?
Answer: _____

4. There are forty-two patients on the ward and six nurses. Each nurse will care for how many patients (assuming each cares for the same number)?
Answer: _____

5. You return your overdue books to the library. The fine is one dollar a day. Three books are two days overdue, and two books are one week overdue. What is your total fine?
Answer: _____

6. A friend agrees to share evenly the library fine (question above) with you. How much will each of you pay?
Answer: _____

7. The budget for a special unit program is $1 100. The total expenses account to $650. (a) How much money remains? (b) What percent of original money remains?
Answers: _____ , _____

8. The bus has forty-two seats. There are fifty people waiting at the bus stop. (a) What fraction of the total will be seated? (b) What fraction of the total will have to stand? (c) What percent will be standing?
Answers: _____ , _____

9. Today — the date isn't important — I went to the corner store — and that isn't important, either — and bought a drink for one dollar, a chocolate bar for two dollars, and a six pack of doughnuts for three dollars and fifty cents. How much did I spend?
Answer: _____

10. The sports store is having a super ski sale. Skis that regularly cost three hundred and ninety-nine dollars now cost one hundred and thirty-seven. How much could you save on a pair of skis?
Answer: _____

11. This week the farmers' market is advertising apples at twenty-five cents each. How much will a dozen cost?
Answer: _____

12. Ten four-year-old children came to the birthday party. There were thirty grab bags, contents unknown. How many could each child have? (One might also ask, how many headaches did the parents have!)
Answer: _____

13. I had two dollars and a craving for licorice. Each stick cost ten cents, and I spent one dollar and sixty cents. How many sticks did I buy, and how much money did I have left?
Answers: _____ , _____

14. The hockey arena sold 14 300 season tickets and 500 single-game tickets. Of these, nine hundred and seventy-eight were sold to nurses. How many "civilians" were at that game?
Answer: _____

15. One box of chocolate bars contains twenty-five bars, at a cost of fifty cents each. What is the total cost of the box?
Answer: _____

16. Forty-five nursing students went to a nightclub to listen to a new comedian. Each table had nine chairs. How many tables did this group need?
Answer: _____

17. Admission to the nightclub is regularly four dollars and fifty cents. If more than one dozen in a group buy tickets, the cost is reduced by fifty cents each. If more than twenty buy tickets, the cost is further reduced by fifty cents. For each additional five individuals in the group, the cost is reduced by twenty-five cents. How much did these enterprising nursing students (question above) each pay to see this comedian?
Answer: _____

18. Your total library fine is five dollars and fifty cents. The fine per day is fifty cents. How many days overdue is your book?
Answer: _____

19. Designer jeans usually priced at one hundred forty-nine dollars and ninety cents have been reduced by nineteen dollars and seventy-five cents. What is the price for the jeans? (Would you want them at this price?)
Answer: _____

YOUR SCORE: _____ %

Systems of Measurement and Abbreviations

Convert each of the following measurements:

1. 10 g = _____ mg

2. 50 mg = _____ g

3. 0.25 g = _____ mg

4. 1.25 mg = _____ micrograms (mcg)

5. 1 L = _____ mL

6. 2 kg = _____ g

7. 350 mg = _____ g

8. 1.5 m = _____ cm

9. 0.7 g = _____ mcg

Convert the following household measurements to SI units:

10. 3.4 fl oz = _____ mL

11. 2 tsp = _____ mL

12. 35 kg = _____ lb

13. 143 lb = _____ kg

Write in full the meaning for each abbreviation:

14. p.c. _____

15. p.r.n. _____

16. stat. _____

17. tab. _____

18. b.i.d. _____

19. h.s. _____

20. ung. _____

21. mg _____

22. mcg _____

23. s.c. _____

24. mEq _____

25. a.c. _____

YOUR SCORE: _____ %

Dosage Calculations

1. Physician orders methyldopa (Aldomet) 500 mg P.O. b.i.d. The medication is available in 250 mg tablets. How many tablets are you required to give?
Answer: _____

2. The medication order for Mrs. Johnson is "erythromycin estolate (Ilosone) 0.5 g P.O. q.12h." The only available dosage is 250 mg tablets. How many tablets do you give to Mrs. Johnson?
Answer: _____

3. A clinical nurse asks you to double check the dosage of insulin. You read the order, which states "regular insulin 15 units and N.P.H. insulin 25 units today." Which syringe indicates the correct dosage?

a.

b.

c.

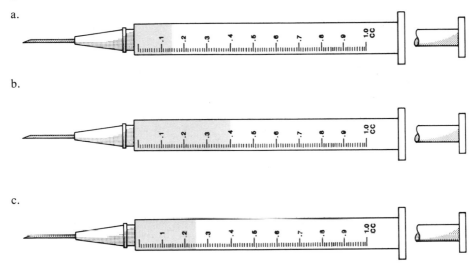

4. Alprazolam (Xanax) 0.25 mg P.O. t.i.d. and 1 mg h.s. is ordered for Mr. Thomson. The drug is available in 0.25 mg tablets. How many are given and when?
Answer: _____

5. Aluminum hydroxide (Amphojel) liquid is requested at 640 mg P.O. q.4h. The available drug is 320 mg/15 mL. (a) How many times is the dosage given in a 24 hour period? (b) How much Amphojel should be given? Indicate the correct amount by shading in the volume below.
Answers: _____ , _____

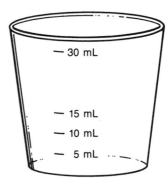

— 30 mL

— 15 mL
— 10 mL
— 5 mL

6. Diphenhydramine HCl (Benadryl) 25 mg I.M. q.6h. p.r.n. is ordered and is available in a 10 mL vial labeled 1 mL = 50 mg. What volume is required to deliver this dosage? Indicate the correct dosage by shading in the volume on the syringe below.

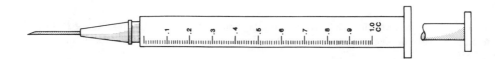

7. The medication order reads "furosemide (Lasix) 30 mg I.V. stat." It is available in a 2 mL ampule containing 20 mg. When and how much is administered? Shade in the correct volume below.

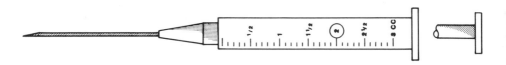

8. Diazepam (Valium) is stocked in a 2 mL ampule containing 10 mg. A preoperative order comes for a patient for 5 mg I.M. What is the correct volume for this dosage?
Answer: _____

9. An I.V. is set up containing 5% dextrose and 0.45% normal saline at 100 mL/hour. The infusion set delivers 60 drops/mL. Calculate the flow rate in drops/minute.
Answer: _____

10. The I.V. in Mr. Sinden's room is infusing at 20 drops/min. The infusion set delivers 10 drops/mL. What is the flow rate in mL/hour?
Answer: _____

11. One unit, 500 mL of whole blood, is to be infused intravenously over the next 4 hours. The drop rate for the blood is 15 drops/mL. What is the flow rate in drops/minute?
Answer: _____

12. The order is for 1 000 mL of I.V. N/S over 8 hours. The drop rate for the N/S is 10 drops/mL. What is the flow rate in drops/minute?
Answer: _____

13. Fifty milliliters of 0.9% sodium chloride is set up in an I.V. to infuse in 20 minutes. The I.V. infusion rate delivers 10 drops/mL. What is the flow rate in drops/minute for this infusion?
Answer: _____

14. Following an initial infusion, a second I.V. is set up for 3 000 mL over 24 hours.
a. What is the flow rate in mL/hour for the I.V.?
b. What is the flow rate in drops/minute if the I.V. set delivers 20 drops/mL?
Answers: _____ , _____

15. A 4-year-old child is to receive digoxin (Lanoxin) 0.02 mg P.O. You find a bottle labeled Lanoxin Elixir 0.05 mg/mL. The dropper is calibrated in tenths of a millilitre. Calculate the amount to administer.
Answer: _____

16. Read the label and then calculate the amount to administer. Give morphine 7 mg I.M.
Answer: _____

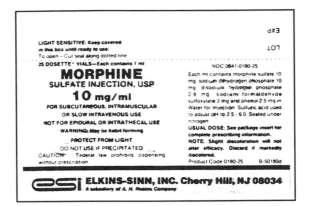

17. Read the label and answer the question.

> LANOXIN
> digoxin
> 250 μg (0.25 mg)

What is the dosage strength of this drug?

1. 250 micrograms/tab.

2. 250 milligrams/tab.

3. 0.25 milligrams/tab.

4. 0.25 micrograms/tab.

  a. 1, 3

  b. 2, 4

18. The label reads nystatin (Mycostatin) oral suspension 100 000 units/mL. The mother just gave 2.5 mL to her child. What dosage of the drug did the child receive?
Answer: _____

Read the labels on p. 10 and answer questions 19 and 20.

19. Which tablet is the greatest dosage strength?
Answer: _____

20. The medication order reads "Synthroid 0.125 mg P.O." How many tablets should you give? State the dosage strength of the tablets.
Answers: _____ , _____

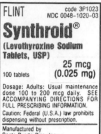

FLINT code 3P1023
NDC 0048-1020-03

Synthroid®

(Levothyroxine Sodium Tablets, USP)

100 tablets

25 mcg
(0.025 mg)

Dosage: Adults: Usual maintenance dose 100 to 200 mcg daily. SEE ACCOMPANYING DIRECTIONS FOR FULL PRESCRIBING INFORMATION.

Caution: Federal (U.S.A.) law prohibits dispensing without prescription.

Manufactured by
Boots Puerto Rico, Inc.
Jayuya, Puerto Rico 00664-0795
For
Flint Laboratories, Inc.
Deerfield, Illinois 60015 U.S.A.

BOOTS-FLINT

100 Tablets code 3P1033
(10 Strips - NDC 0048-1040-13
10 Unit Dose tablets each)

SYNTHROID®

(Levothyroxine Sodium Tablets, USP)

50 mcg (0.05 mg)

Dosage: Adults: Initial - 25 to 100 mcg (0.025 to 0.1 mg) daily. Usual mainte-nance dose - 100 to 200 mcg (0.1 to 0.2 mg) daily. Children: Initial - 25 mcg (0.025 mg) daily. Dosage adjusted by physician until desired response is ob-tained. See directions for higher main-tenance dosage. SEE ACCOMPANYING DIRECTIONS.

Keep this and all medications out of the reach of children.

For hospital use only: Packaging is not child resistant.

Caution: Federal (U.S.A.) law prohibits dispensing without prescription.

Manufactured by Boots Puerto Rico, Inc.
Jayuya, Puerto Rico 00664-0795
For Boots-Flint, Inc.
Lincolnshire, IL 60015 USA
a subsidiary of
The Boots Company (USA) Inc.
13-1040-02
11/87

BOOTS-FLINT

100 Tablets code 3P1003
(10 Strips - NDC 0048-1050-13
10 Unit Dose tablets each)

SYNTHROID®

(Levothyroxine Sodium Tablets, USP)

75 mcg (0.075 mg)

Dosage: Adults: Initial - 25 to 100 mcg (0.025 to 0.1 mg) daily. Usual mainte-nance dose - 100 to 200 mcg (0.1 to 0.2 mg) daily. Children: Initial - 25 mcg (0.025 mg) daily. Dosage adjusted by physician until desired response is ob-tained. See directions for higher main-tenance dosage. SEE ACCOMPANYING DIRECTIONS.

Keep this and all medications out of the reach of children.

For hospital use only: Packaging is not child resistant.

Caution: Federal (U.S.A.) law prohibits dispensing without prescription.

Manufactured by Boots Puerto Rico, Inc.
Jayuya, Puerto Rico 00664-0795
For Boots-Flint, Inc.
Lincolnshire, IL 60015 USA
a subsidiary of
The Boots Company (USA) Inc.
13-1050-02
11/87

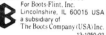

YOUR SCORE: _____ %

Diagnose Your Strengths and Weaknesses

	Number of questions	Your score
Arithmetic of whole numbers	16	
Arithmetic of fractions	21	
Arithmetic of decimal numbers	20	
Word problems	19	
Systems of measurement and abbreviations	25	
Dosage calculations	20	

TOTAL: 121 = 100%

Module 2: Fractions

PRETEST

Instructions

1. Write the pretest without referring to any resources.

2. Express all fractions in their lowest terms (simplified).

3. Correct the pretest using the answer guide.

4. If your score is 100 percent, proceed to the next module.

5. If you don't achieve 100 percent accuracy, read the learning package in this module and complete the exercises, concentrating on your weak areas, as diagnosed by your pretest score.

Addition of Fractions

1. $\frac{2}{5} + 3\frac{1}{4} =$

2. $\frac{1}{3} + \frac{7}{10} + \frac{1}{5} =$

3. $2 + \frac{3}{4} =$

4. $3\frac{1}{8} + 4\frac{1}{6} =$

5. $\frac{2}{3} + \frac{6}{7} =$

6. $\frac{21}{32} + \frac{5}{16} =$

7. $\frac{9}{16} + \frac{3}{8} =$

Subtraction of Fractions

8. $\frac{7}{8} - \frac{2}{9} =$

9. $1\frac{1}{4} - \frac{3}{5} =$

10. $3 - \frac{7}{16} =$

11. $9\frac{3}{8} - 6\frac{7}{16} =$

12. $\dfrac{3}{7} - \dfrac{1}{4} =$

13. $\dfrac{5}{9} - \dfrac{7}{16} =$

14. $\dfrac{5}{8} - \dfrac{3}{5} =$

Multiplication of Fractions

15. $\dfrac{2}{3} \times \dfrac{3}{4} =$

16. $3\dfrac{1}{4} \times 4\dfrac{1}{2} =$

17. $16 \times \dfrac{3}{10} =$

18. $3\dfrac{1}{2} \times 9 =$

19. $2 \times \dfrac{5}{8} =$

20. $\dfrac{7}{16} \times \dfrac{3}{7} =$

21. $10\dfrac{1}{4} \times \dfrac{1}{2} =$

Division of Fractions

22. $\dfrac{16}{27} \div \dfrac{2}{3} =$

23. $1\dfrac{1}{2} \div \dfrac{1}{2} =$

24. $76 \div \dfrac{3}{4} =$

25. $\dfrac{9}{16} \div 3 =$

26. $100 \div \dfrac{3}{4} =$

27. $2\dfrac{3}{4} \div \dfrac{1}{8} =$

28. $\dfrac{7}{16} \div \dfrac{3}{7} =$

Change These Improper Fractions to Mixed or Whole Numbers

29. $\dfrac{18}{5} =$

30. $\dfrac{83}{11} =$

31. $\dfrac{49}{6} =$

32. $\dfrac{127}{34} =$

33. $\dfrac{39}{8} =$

34. $\dfrac{125}{12} =$

Find the Lowest Common Denominator

35. $\dfrac{1}{2}$ and $\dfrac{1}{4}$

36. $\dfrac{1}{5}$ and $\dfrac{1}{6}$

37. $\dfrac{5}{8}$ and $\dfrac{2}{5}$

38. $\dfrac{2}{3}$ and $\dfrac{7}{8}$

Simplify These Fractions to Their Lowest Terms

39. $\dfrac{21}{24} =$

40. $\dfrac{18}{72} =$

41. $\dfrac{6}{9} =$

42. $\dfrac{15}{35} =$

43. $\dfrac{20}{32} =$

44. $\dfrac{5}{75} =$

Identify the Following Expressions as Proper or Improper Fractions or Mixed Numbers

45. $\dfrac{7}{15}$

46. $\dfrac{21}{11}$

47. $1\dfrac{7}{8}$

48. $\dfrac{1}{30}$

49. $\dfrac{1}{17}$ 50. $\dfrac{6}{7}$

51. $3\dfrac{1}{10}$ 52. $\dfrac{9}{5}$

Equivalent Fractions

Express each fraction as an equivalent fraction.

53. $\dfrac{1}{2} = \dfrac{?}{6}$ 54. $\dfrac{3}{20} = \dfrac{9}{?}$

55. $\dfrac{7}{9} = \dfrac{?}{27}$ 56. $\dfrac{7}{10} = \dfrac{49}{?}$

57. $\dfrac{1}{5} = \dfrac{6}{?}$

Are the following expressions equivalent fractions?

58. $\dfrac{3}{8} = \dfrac{15}{30}$ Yes or No

59. $\dfrac{21}{30} = \dfrac{126}{180}$ Yes or No

Change to Improper Fractions

60. $6\dfrac{1}{8} =$

61. $7\dfrac{9}{10} =$

62. $5\dfrac{1}{2} =$

Word Problems

63. There are thirty-six students in the class. One-half achieved a B grade and another quarter achieved honors. The remaining students failed the exam. How many students failed the exam?
Answer: _____

64. A pie was divided into eighths. One individual ate one piece; a second individual ate three pieces. How much of the pie is left?
Answer: _____

65. In a survey of seventy-two people, one-sixth preferred brand X and seven-eighteenths preferred brand Y. The remainder chose brand Z. How many chose brand Z?
Answer: _____

66. In an election, one-fourth of the voters liked candidate Smith, five-eighths disliked the candidate. How many voters were undecided?
Answer: _____

67. A bottle of liquid contains thirty ounces. Every day, one-fifth of the liquid is used. How much liquid remains after the third day?
Answer: _____

68. You have two cups of liquid including one-quarter cup of water, one-fifth cup of syrup, and a secret ingredient. What is the amount of the secret ingredient?
Answer: _____

YOUR SCORE: _____ %

100%   YES — proceed to the next module
        NO — review this module

_____

Note: if you had any errors on this pretest, analyze your areas of weakness.

Learning Package

> ## Objective
> To demonstrate 100 percent accuracy in the arithmetic skills of addition, subtraction, multiplication, and division of mixed numbers and fractions

Definitions

The word *fraction* is from the Latin fractus, meaning "broken." A fraction is a number that represents a part of a whole unit.

The *numerator* is the top value. The *denominator* is the bottom value. **Example:** in $\frac{3}{4}$ the numerator is 3, the denominator is 4.

Types of Fractions

Proper: the numerator is less in value than the denominator: for example, $\frac{1}{3}$

Improper fraction: the numerator is greater in value than the denominator: for example, $\frac{4}{3}$

Mixed number: a unit contains a whole number and a fraction: for example, $1\frac{1}{3}$

Equivalent fractions: fractions have the same value but are expressed in different forms. A fraction can have both terms — numerator and denominator — multiplied by the same number without changing its value. Likewise, both terms of a fraction can be divided by the same number without changing its value. This is an important principle in the arithmetic of fractions.

$$\frac{1\,(\times 2)}{2\,(\times 2)} = \frac{2}{4}$$

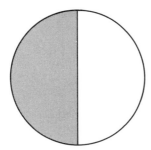
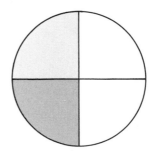

Lowest term: the numerator and denominator have the lowest possible value. This is accomplished by dividing the denominator and the numerator by the same number.

Example: $\frac{1}{2}$ is in its lowest term.

$\frac{2}{4}$ is not expressed in its lowest term.

It can be simplified by:
1. Dividing both the numerator and the denominator by the same number, in this example, by 2.
2. Placing the new value of the numerator over the new value of the denominator

$$\frac{2}{4} = \frac{?}{?}$$

$$\frac{2\,(\div\,2)}{4\,(\div\,2)} = \frac{1}{2}$$

Equivalent fraction in lowest term is $\frac{1}{2}$

Changing Improper Fractions and Mixed Numbers

An *improper fraction* can be changed to a *mixed number* by dividing the numerator by the denominator.

Example: $\frac{4}{3} = 1\frac{1}{3}$

$$4 \div 3 = 1\frac{1}{3}$$

Similarly, a *mixed number* may be changed to an *improper fraction* by:

1. Multiplying the whole number by the denominator.

2. Adding the numerator to the product.

3. Placing the sum over the denominator.

Example: $5\frac{1}{3} = ?$

$$\frac{5 \times 3 + 1}{3} = \frac{16}{3}$$

$$\text{because } 5 = \frac{15}{3}$$

$$\frac{15}{3} + \frac{1}{3} = \frac{16}{3}$$

Arithmetic of Fractions

Adding Fractions

To add fractions with the same denominator:

1. Add the numerators.

2. Place the sum over the denominator.

3. Simplify if necessary.

$$\text{Example: } \frac{1}{5} + \frac{2}{5}$$

$$\frac{1+2}{5} = \frac{3}{5}$$

To add fractions with unlike denominators:

1. Find the common denominator. This is the smallest whole number that the denominators of two or more fractions will divide into evenly.

2. Convert each fraction to an equivalent fraction using the common denominator.

3. Add numerators and place the sum over the common denominator.

4. Simplify the answer.

$$\text{Example: } \frac{1}{2} + \frac{2}{3} = ?$$

Common denominator is 6: both 2 and 3 divide evenly into this number.

$$\text{Convert: } \frac{1\,(\times 3)}{2\,(\times 3)} = \frac{3}{6}$$

$$\frac{2\,(\times 2)}{3\,(\times 2)} = \frac{4}{6}$$

$$\text{Add: } \frac{3}{6} + \frac{4}{6} = \frac{3+4}{6} = \frac{7}{6}$$

$$\text{Simplify: } \frac{7}{6} = 1\frac{1}{6}$$

Subtracting Fractions

To subtract fractions that have the same denominator:

1. Subtract the numerators.

2. Place the answer over the denominator.

3. Simplify if necessary.

These steps are illustrated in the following example.

$$\text{Example: } \frac{3}{4} - \frac{1}{4} = ?$$

$$\frac{3-1}{4} = \frac{2}{4} = \frac{1}{2}$$

To subtract fractions with unlike denominators:

1. Find the common denominator.

2. Convert each fraction to an equivalent fraction using the common denominator.

3. Subtract the numerators and place the difference over the common denominator.

4. Simplify if necessary.

$$\text{Example: } \frac{5}{6} - \frac{3}{8} = ?$$

The common denominator is 24

$$\text{Convert: } \frac{5}{6} = \frac{?}{24} \qquad \frac{5(\times 4)}{6(\times 4)} = \frac{20}{24}$$

$$\text{Convert: } \frac{3}{8} = \frac{?}{24} \qquad \frac{3(\times 3)}{8(\times 3)} = \frac{9}{24}$$

$$\text{Subtract: } \frac{20-9}{24} = \frac{11}{24}$$

$$\text{Simplify: } \frac{11}{24} \text{ is expressed in the lowest term}$$

Adding and Subtracting Mixed Numbers

To add or subtract mixed numbers, first convert the mixed number to an improper fraction, then follow the steps outlined for addition and subtraction of fractions.

Example: $1\dfrac{1}{3} + \dfrac{3}{4} = ?$

Convert the mixed number:

$1\dfrac{1}{3}$ is $\dfrac{4}{3}$

Find the common denominator:
12 is evenly divided by both 3 and 4

Convert: $\dfrac{4\,(\times 4)}{3\,(\times 4)} = \dfrac{16}{12}$

Convert: $\dfrac{3\,(\times 3)}{4\,(\times 3)} = \dfrac{9}{12}$

$\dfrac{16 + 9}{12} = \dfrac{25}{12}$

Convert to mixed number: $\dfrac{25}{12} = 2\,\dfrac{1}{12}$

Example: $2 - \dfrac{1}{2} = ?$

Convert the whole number to a fraction:

$2 = \dfrac{2}{1}$

Find the common denominator: 2

Convert: $\dfrac{2\,(\times 2)}{1\,(\times 2)} = \dfrac{4}{2}$

Subtract: $\dfrac{4 - 1}{2} = \dfrac{3}{2}$

Convert to mixed number: $\dfrac{3}{2} = 1\,\dfrac{1}{2}$

To add or subtract mixed numbers, you may also follow this example:

Example: $2\frac{1}{2} + 3\frac{1}{3}$

Add the whole numbers: $2 + 3 = 5$

Add the fractions: $\frac{1}{2} + \frac{1}{3}$

Convert to a common denominator:

$$\frac{1\,(\times 3)}{2\,(\times 3)} = \frac{3}{6}$$

$$\frac{1\,(\times 2)}{3\,(\times 2)} = \frac{2}{6}$$

Add the fractions: $\frac{3 + 2}{6} = \frac{5}{6}$

Add to the whole number: $5\frac{5}{6}$

Multiplication of Fractions

To multiply fractions:

1. Multiply the numerators.

2. Multiply the denominators.

3. Place the product of the numerator over the product of the denominators.

4. Simplify if necessary.

Example: $\frac{2}{3} \times \frac{5}{7}$

$$\frac{2 \times 5}{3 \times 7} = \frac{10}{21}$$

To multiply a fraction by a whole number:

1. Multiply only the numerator of the fraction by the whole number.

2. Place the product over the denominator.

3. Simplify if necessary, or express the whole number as a fraction and proceed as outlined.

Example: $5 \times \frac{3}{7} = ?$

$$\frac{5}{1} \times \frac{3}{7} = \frac{5 \times 3}{1 \times 7} = \frac{15}{7}$$

Simplify: $\frac{15}{7} = 2\frac{1}{7}$

To multiply a fraction by a mixed number:

1. Change it to an improper fraction.

2. Multiply the numerators.

3. Multiply the denominators.

4. Place the product of the numerators over the product of the denominators.

5. Simplify if necessary or convert to mixed number.

Example: $3\frac{1}{5} \times \frac{3}{4} = ?$

$$3\frac{1}{5} = \frac{16}{5}$$

$$\frac{16}{5} \times \frac{3}{4} = \frac{16 \times 3}{5 \times 4} = \frac{48}{20}$$

Simplify: $\frac{48}{20} = 2\frac{2}{5}$

Division of Fractions

To divide fractions:

1. Invert the terms of the *divisor*. This is the number that is being divided into the *dividend*.

2. Then use multiplication.

Example: $\frac{1}{3} \div \frac{1}{2} = ?$

Invert the divisor: $\frac{1}{2} = \frac{2}{1}$

Multiply: $\frac{1}{3} \times \frac{2}{1} = \frac{1 \times 2}{3 \times 1} = \frac{2}{3}$

To divide a fraction by a whole number:

1. Express the whole number as a fraction.

2. Invert the divisor.

3. Use multiplication.

4. Simplify or convert to mixed number.

Example: $\dfrac{5}{6} \div 2 = ?$

2 as a fraction is $\dfrac{2}{1}$

Invert: $\dfrac{2}{1}$ becomes $\dfrac{1}{2}$

Multiply: $\dfrac{5}{6} \times \dfrac{1}{2} = \dfrac{5 \times 1}{6 \times 2} = \dfrac{5}{12}$

To divide a fraction by a mixed number:

1. Change the mixed number to an improper fraction.

2. Invert the divisor.

3. Use multiplication.

4. Simplify if necessary.

Example: $\dfrac{3}{4} \div 1\dfrac{1}{8} = ?$

Convert to improper fraction:

$1\dfrac{1}{8} = \dfrac{9}{8}$

Invert the divisor: $\dfrac{9}{8} = \dfrac{8}{9}$

Multiply: $\dfrac{3}{4} \times \dfrac{8}{9} = \dfrac{3 \times 8}{4 \times 9} = \dfrac{24}{36}$

Simplify: $\dfrac{24\,(\div 12)}{36\,(\div 12)} = \dfrac{2}{3}$

POSTTEST

Instructions

1. Write the posttest without referring to any reference materials.

2. Express all fractions in their lowest terms.

3. Correct the posttest using the answer guide.

4. If your score is 100 percent, proceed to the next module.

5. If you don't achieve 100 percent, analyze your problems and review the appropriate sections of the learning package in this module. Then rewrite the posttest.

Addition of Fractions

1. $\dfrac{3}{4} + \dfrac{1}{7} =$

2. $\dfrac{1}{8} + 1\dfrac{2}{5} =$

3. $\dfrac{3}{7} + \dfrac{1}{2} =$

4. $14 + \dfrac{7}{12} =$

5. $\dfrac{5}{12} + \dfrac{2}{10} =$

6. $\dfrac{5}{9} + \dfrac{15}{18} =$

Subtraction of Fractions

7. $\dfrac{8}{9} - \dfrac{5}{12} =$

8. $2\dfrac{1}{2} - \dfrac{1}{6} =$

9. $4\dfrac{1}{5} - 3 =$

10. $21 - \dfrac{15}{16} =$

11. $\dfrac{7}{8} - \dfrac{2}{3} =$

12. $\dfrac{11}{15} - \dfrac{3}{8} =$

Multiplication of Fractions

13. $\dfrac{2}{9} \times \dfrac{3}{7} =$

14. $1\dfrac{1}{2} \times \dfrac{2}{5} =$

15. $\dfrac{3}{4} \times 100 =$

16. $23 \times \dfrac{1}{3} =$

17. $\dfrac{3}{4} \times 4 =$

18. $1\dfrac{1}{2} \times 52 =$

Division of Fractions

19. $\frac{9}{16} \div \frac{3}{4} =$

20. $3\frac{1}{4} \div \frac{1}{3} =$

21. $\frac{9}{15} \div \frac{2}{3} =$

22. $\frac{5}{6} \div 2 =$

23. $\frac{5}{9} \div \frac{7}{10} =$

24. $10 \div \frac{3}{4} =$

Express as Improper Fractions

25. $12\frac{2}{3} =$

26. $3\frac{2}{4} =$

Change These Improper Fractions to Mixed or Whole Numbers

27. $\frac{21}{5} =$

28. $\frac{38}{9} =$

29. $\frac{11}{4} =$

30. $\frac{89}{7} =$

31. $\frac{203}{12} =$

32. $\frac{10}{3} =$

Find the Lowest Common Denominator

33. $\frac{7}{9}$ and $\frac{3}{8}$

34. $\frac{15}{16}$ and $\frac{2}{3}$

35. $\frac{13}{18}$ and $\frac{23}{24}$

36. $\frac{5}{6}$ and $\frac{4}{7}$

Reduce to the Lowest Terms

37. $\dfrac{16}{36} =$

38. $\dfrac{25}{45} =$

39. $\dfrac{15}{18} =$

40. $\dfrac{12}{4} =$

41. Which of the following is a proper fraction? Circle your choice.

$$\dfrac{8}{9} \qquad \dfrac{4}{3} \qquad 1\dfrac{1}{4}$$

42. Which of the following is an improper fraction? Circle your choice.

$$\dfrac{7}{8} \qquad \dfrac{21}{30} \qquad \dfrac{14}{11}$$

43. Which of the following is a mixed number? Circle your choice.

$$1\dfrac{2}{3} \qquad \dfrac{7}{7} \qquad \dfrac{5}{9}$$

Express the Following Fractions as Equivalent Fractions

44. $\dfrac{5}{7} = \dfrac{35}{?}$

45. $\dfrac{14}{35} = \dfrac{28}{?}$

46. $\dfrac{5}{9} = \dfrac{?}{108}$

47. $\dfrac{3}{20} = \dfrac{?}{200}$

48. $\dfrac{8}{11} = \dfrac{32}{?}$

Word Problems

49. Of thirty people, $\frac{8}{30}$ like skiing, $\frac{5}{30}$ like fishing, and the remaining don't like any sports. Expressed as a whole number, how many individuals would rather do something else?
Answer: _____

50. A bottle of aspirin contains one hundred pills. If sixteen friends had simultaneous headaches and half of them took two pills each, and one-quarter took one pill each, how many aspirin would remain?
Answer: _____

51. If you attend a two-hour lecture and spend five-sixths of the time taking notes, how many minutes do you rest your hand?
Answer: _____

52. Of forty-five students in class, one-ninth fell asleep. How many stayed awake for the lecture?
Answer: _____

53. One of the students answered the following question:

$$\frac{4}{5} \times \frac{3}{2} = ? \qquad \text{Answer:} \frac{8}{15}$$

Is this answer correct?   Yes or No
(I won't ask whether you think this student stayed awake during class!)

54. You have just completed the second of ten modules. Express that as a fraction.
Answer: _____

YOUR SCORE: _____ %

100%   YES—proceed to the next module
NO —review this module

Note: if you had any errors on the posttest, analyze your areas of weakness before reviewing the module.

Module 3: Decimal Numbers

PRETEST

Instructions

1. Write the pretest without referring to any resources.

2. Correct the pretest using the answer guide.

3. If your score is 100 percent, proceed to the next module.

4. If you don't achieve 100 percent accuracy, read the learning package in this module and complete the exercises, concentrating on your weak areas as diagnosed by your pretest score.

Note: be careful to write the decimal numbers correctly — according to the rules — and do *not* round any numbers unless instructed to do so.

For each of the following pairs, choose the correct way of writing decimals. Circle your choice.

1. .25 or 0.25   2. 1.0 or 1

3. 0.120 or 0.12

Rounding Decimal Numbers

Round the following decimal numbers to the nearest tenth.

4. 3.43   5. 7.09

6. 1.239   7. 9.16

Round the following decimal numbers to the nearest hundredth.

8. 12.459   9. 6.096

10. 34.002   11. 4.909

Addition of Decimal Numbers

12. $1.567 + 0.98 =$

13. $123.5 + 2.534\ 2 =$

14. $0.4 + 5.6 + 0.27 =$

15. $2.1 + 0.53 + 1.102 =$

Subtraction of Decimal Numbers

16. $10 - 3.7 =$

17. $4.2 - 0.9 =$

18. $5.6 - 1.08 =$

19. $0.125 - 0.075 =$

Multiplication of Decimal Numbers

20. $0.8 \times 10 =$

21. $0.8 \times 100 =$

22. $0.8 \times 1\ 000 =$

23. $0.1 \times 0.01 =$

Division of Decimal Numbers

24. $0.25 \div 0.5 =$

25. $100 \div 1.5 -$

26. $0.667 \div 0.3 =$

27. $1.78 \div 0.04 =$

Convert into Decimal Numbers. Round to the Nearest Tenth

28. $\dfrac{4}{5} =$

29. $\dfrac{1}{2} =$

30. $\dfrac{1}{4} =$

31. $\dfrac{3}{4} =$

Convert into Fractions. Simplify to Lowest Terms

32. $0.6 =$

33. $0.57 =$

34. $1.25 =$

35. $0.01 =$

Arrange in Size from Smallest to Largest

36. 0.01   0.000 1   0.1   1.001   1.101

Word Problems

37. John had $0.40 and Susan had twice as much money as John. In total, how much money did they have?
Answer: _____

38. A baseball glove costs $36.95. David has $48.65. How much will he have left after he buys the glove?
Answer: _____

39. A soccer team won the game and the coach bought pizzas. She ordered twelve pizzas and each cost $7.95. How much did she pay?
Answer: _____

40. Together, four girls earned $45.48. How much did each girl earn?
Answer: _____

YOUR SCORE: _____ %

100%   YES—proceed to the next module
NO —complete this module

Note: if you had any errors on the pretest, analyze your areas of weakness.

Learning Package

> **Objective**
> To demonstrate 100 percent accuracy in the arithmetic skills of addition, subtraction, multiplication, and division of decimal numbers, and in converting decimal numbers, percents, and fractions

Decimal numbers express values that describe both whole units and portions of whole units. Decimal numbers include a decimal point and values to the right and left of the decimal. The numbers written to the left of the decimal point are whole numbers. The numbers written to the right of the decimal point are decimal fractions, that is, fractions with denominators in multiples of ten. Thus:

$$0.1 = \frac{1}{10} \text{ or one-tenth}$$

$$0.01 = \frac{1}{100} \text{ or one-hundredth}$$

$$0.001 = \frac{1}{1\,000} \text{ or one-thousandth}$$

> Example: In the number 6.125 there are:
>
> 6 ones
>
> $\frac{1}{10}$ or one tenth
>
> $\frac{2}{100}$ or two-hundredths
>
> $\frac{5}{1\,000}$ or five-thousandths

The size of decimal numbers can be compared by examining the values in each position to the right and left of the decimal point.

> Example: Which is larger, 0.5 or 0.05?
>
> 0 ones   0.5   5 tenths
>
> 0 ones   0.05   0 tenths, 5 hundredths
>
> Therefore, 0.5 is larger than 0.05

Rules for Writing Decimal Numbers

1. Always place a zero to the left of the decimal point when there are no whole numbers.

> Example: 0.25, not .25

2. Never place a zero to the right of the decimal point.

> Example: 1, not 1.0
> 1.2, not 1.20

These rules are extremely important when writing drug dosages. If a drug is ordered as 0.125 mg, the zero placed before the decimal highlights the point that might otherwise be missed. If 0.125 mg is misread as 125 mg, a fatal drug error could occur. Similarly, the zero placed after the decimal point is unnecessary. A drug order for 6 units is less likely to be misinterpreted than one written as 6.0 units. Missing the point could cause a tenfold error.

3. As with whole numbers, spaces are used to separate decimal numbers into three-digit blocks.

> Example: 1.000 1
> 1.078 35

Rounding Decimal Numbers

Most calibrated devices used for medication administration are accurate only to the nearest tenth or hundredth. Consequently, it is acceptable to round dosage calculations to significant digits.

To round a decimal number:

1. Locate the digit furthest to the right of the decimal point.

2. If this digit is 5 or greater, add a value of 1 to the numeral to its immediate left.

3. If this digit is less than 5, do not increase the value of the numeral to its immediate left.

4. Continue this process one digit at a time, moving right to left toward the decimal point.

> Example: Round 1.125 to the nearest hundredth.
>   The digit in the hundredth position is 2.
>   The digit to the right is 5.
>   Increase the value of the numeral in the hundredth place by 1.
> Answer: 1.13
>
> Round 1.125 to the nearest tenth.
>   The digit in the tenth position is 1.
>   The digit to the right is 2.
>   Do not add value to the tenth.
> Answer: 1.1

Exercise 3.1

Complete the following exercise without referring to the previous text. Correct using the answer guide.

Some of the following decimal numbers violate the rules. Correct those that don't follow the rules.

1. 1.02   2. 1.70

3. 0.67   4. .35

Round these decimal numbers to the nearest tenth:

5. 1.362   6. 1.94

7. 0.99   8. 1.07

Round these decimal numbers to the nearest hundredth:

9. 6.333 5   10. 2.090 9

11. 0.951   12. 7.666

13. Arrange the following in order from smallest to largest:

    1.15   1.105   1.055   1.515

14. Arrange the following in order from largest to smallest:

            5.06   50.6   0.506

Arithmetic of Decimal Numbers

Addition and Subtraction of Decimal Numbers

Decimal points must be lined up vertically, so that tenths are under tenths, hundredths under hundredths, etc.

Addition	Subtraction
Example: 1.9 + 0.37 + 2.706	Example: 2.75 − 0.59
1.9	2.75
0.37	−0.59
2.706	2.16
4.976	

Exercise 3.2

Complete the following exercise without referring to the previous text. Correct using the answer guide.

1. $3.51 + 2.03 + 0.9 =$

2. $10.1 + 3.27 + 1.003 =$

3. $27.3 - 16.09 =$

4. $5.03 - 3.27 =$

5. $0.056 + 1.990\ 1 =$

6. $40\ 076.5 - 1.679\ 3 =$

Multiplication of Decimal Numbers

The multiplication of decimal numbers follows the same rules as those for the multiplication of whole numbers. To determine the placement of the decimal point:

1. Count the number of digits to the right of the decimal point in each of the numbers being multiplied.

2. Add these numbers.

3. Place the decimal with this number of digits to the right of the decimal point.

Example: $2.162 \times 13.4 = ?$

2.162: 3 digits to the right of the decimal
13.4: 1 digit to the right of the decimal

The answer must have 4 digits to the right of the decimal point.

$$
\begin{array}{r}
2.162 \\
\times\ 13.4 \\
\hline
8648 \\
6486 \\
2162 \\
\hline
289708
\end{array}
$$

Place decimal point with 4 digits to the right: 28.970 8

Division of Decimal Numbers

To divide decimal numbers:

1. Write the problem as you would for the division of whole numbers.

2. Move the decimal place to the right in the divisor, so that it becomes a whole number. This is achieved by multiplying 10, 100, 1 000, etc.

3. Move the decimal point the same number of positions to the right in the dividend; that is, multiply both the divisor and the dividend by 10, 100, 1 000, etc.

4. Place decimal directly above the decimal in the dividend.

Example: 2.5 $\overline{)\ 12.55}$ = ?

Divisor is 2.5
Dividend is 12.55
Multiply both the divisor and the dividend by 10; that is, move the decimal point one place to the right in *both* numbers.

$$25 \overline{)\ \begin{array}{r} 5.02 \\ 125.5 \\ \underline{125} \\ 0.5 \\ \underline{0.50} \\ .00 \end{array}}$$

$$\frac{12.55 \times 10}{2.5\ \ \times 10} = \frac{125.5}{25}$$

$$25 \overline{)\ 125.5}$$

decimal placed directly above

Exercise 3.3

Complete the following exercise without referring to the previous text. Correct using the answer guide.

1. 1.27×3.2 =

2. 2.73×1.4 =

3. 10.078×0.34 =

4. $1.900\ 1 \times 30.6$ =

5. $1.29 \div 0.3$ =

6. $17.588 \div 0.02$ =

7. $0.25 \div 0.5$ =

8. $1\ 000.25 \div 0.001$ =

Converting Fractions and Decimal Numbers

To convert a fraction to a decimal number, divide the numerator by the denominator.

Example: $\frac{1}{2}$ = ?

$1 \div 2 = 0.5$

To convert a decimal number to a fraction:

1. Determine the denominator as 10, 100, 1 000, etc. by the number of digits to the right of the decimal point.

2. Express as a fraction by placing the number over the selected denominator.

3. Simplify if necessary.

Example: 0.6 has 1 digit to the right

$$= \text{tenths or } \frac{6}{10}$$

0.06 has 2 digits to the right

$$= \text{hundredths or } \frac{6}{100}$$

0.006 has 3 digits to the right

$$= \text{thousandths or } \frac{6}{1\ 000}$$

Example: Convert 0.06 to a fraction
Denominator is 100

$$\frac{6}{100} = \frac{3}{50}$$

Value Chart

Decimal	Tenths	Hundredths	Thousandths
	6		
	0	6	
	0	0	6

To convert a mixed number to a decimal number:

1. Express the mixed number as an improper fraction.

2. Divide the numerator by the denominator.

Example: $1\frac{1}{4} = ?$

$1\frac{1}{4} = \frac{5}{4}$

$$\begin{array}{r} 1.25 \\ 4\,\overline{)\,5.00} \\ \underline{4} \\ 10 \\ \underline{8} \\ 20 \\ \underline{20} \end{array}$$

Exercise 3.4

Complete the following exercise without referring to the previous text. Correct using the answer guide.

Convert the following decimal numbers to proper or mixed fractions and express in lowest terms:

1. $0.125 =$

2. $2.5 =$

3. $0.6 =$

4. $0.75 =$

5. $1.75 =$

Convert the following fractions to decimal numbers. Be certain to use a zero to the left of the decimal point where necessary.

6. $\frac{3}{4} =$

7. $\frac{1}{20} =$

8. $3\frac{5}{6} =$

9. $\frac{1}{3}$

10. $1\frac{1}{4} =$

Percent

Percent means "parts in a hundred." $\frac{N}{100} = N\%$. Our most frequent encounter with percentages is with relation to exam scores. For example, if your score is 90 percent, you answered 90 questions out of 100 correctly. However, few exams have 100 questions—thankfully! What does percent mean when there are only 30 rather than 100 parts? The first step is to convert to an equivalent fraction. If you answered 12 questions correctly out of 30, your score would be:

Example: Express as equivalent fraction

$$\frac{12}{30} = \frac{N}{100}$$

Solve: 30N = 1200

$$N = \frac{1200}{30} = 30 \overline{)\ 1200}^{\ 40}$$
$$\underline{1200}$$

Add percent sign = 40%

Your score is 40%.

To change a decimal number to a percent:

1. Multiply the decimal by 100.

2. Add the % sign.

Example: 0.67 = ?

0.67 × 100 = 67

67%

To change a fraction to a percent:

1. Convert the fraction to a decimal number (previously explained in this module).

2. Multiply the decimal by 100.

3. Add the % sign.

Example: $\frac{1}{5}$ = ?

$\frac{1}{5} = 0.2$

0.2 × 100 = 20

20%

To change a percent to a decimal number:

1. Remove the percent sign.

2. Divide by 100.

3. Write the decimal number according to the rules.

Example: 40% = ?

40

40 ÷ 100 = .4

0.4

To change a percent to a fraction:

1. Place percent number over 100.

2. Simplify if necessary.

Example: 40% = ?

$$\frac{40}{100} = \frac{2}{5}$$

Exercise 3.5

Complete the following exercise without referring to the previous text. Correct using the answer guide.

Express these decimal numbers as percents:

1. 1.5 =   2. 0.37 =

3. 0.17 =   4. 0.94 =

Express these fractions as percents:

5. $\dfrac{1}{15}$ =   6. $\dfrac{25}{30}$ =

7. $\dfrac{8}{11}$ =   8. $\dfrac{79}{100}$ =

Express these percents as decimal numbers:

9. 77% =   10. 1% =

11. 29% =   12. 82% =

Express these percents as fractions:

13. 25% =   14. 33% =

15. 6% =   16. 12.5% =

POSTTEST

Instructions

1. Write the posttest without referring to any reference materials.

2. Unless instructed otherwise, round decimal numbers to the nearest hundredth.

3. Correct the posttest using the answer guide.

4. If your score is 100 percent, proceed to the next module.

5. If you don't achieve 100 percent accuracy, review the appropriate sections of the learning package in this module and rewrite the posttest. You may want to complete the additional exercises in Appendix A.

Addition of Decimal Numbers

1. $1.347 + 2.8 =$ 2. $0.069 + 1.7 =$

3. $1.21 + 0.05 =$ 4. $1.239 + 0.08 =$

Subtraction of Decimal Numbers

5. $3.52 - 1.19 =$ 6. $8.57 - 6.68 =$

7. $18.09 - 16.9 =$ 8. $3.43 - 1.009\ 7 =$

Multiplication of Decimal Numbers

9. $5.06 \times 2.1 =$ 10. $10.1 \times 0.03 =$

11. $2.5 \times 1.7 =$ 12. $1.01 \times 100 =$

Division of Decimal Numbers

13. $9 \div 0.05 =$ 14. $0.25 \div 2 =$

15. $0.1 \div 0.05 =$ 16. $12.3 \div 4.1 =$

Rounding Decimal Numbers

Round to the nearest tenth.

17. 4.15   18. 1.77

19. 1.26   20. 2.33

Round to the nearest hundredth.

21. 1.885   22. 1.973

23. 10.635   24. 0.359

Converting Decimal Numbers

Convert these fractions to decimal numbers.

25. $\frac{2}{3}$ =   26. $1\frac{1}{4}$ =

27. $\frac{7}{8}$ =   28. $2\frac{1}{2}$ =

Convert these decimal numbers to fractions and simplify.

29. 0.76 =   30. 1.3 =

31. 0.13 =   32. 0.05 =

Indicate which of the following correctly express the decimal number according to the rules. Circle your choice.

33. $\frac{1}{2}$ = .5 or 0.5   34. 1.2 or 1.20

35. 1.010 or 1.01

Arrange in size from smallest to largest.

36. 10.01   1.901   10.1   1.991

Word Problems

37. James had $437.62 in his bank account. He earned $13.46 and deposited it in the bank. What is his current bank balance?
Answer: _____

38. Jodi wanted to withdraw $18.25 from her bank account to purchase a photo album. She had $405.02 in the account. What is her balance after the withdrawal?
Answer: _____

39. Dave bought twenty-eight eggs at $0.14 each. How much did he spend?
Answer: _____

40. For the fiscal year 1988–1989 a company's profits were $22 139.88. If there are forty-two employees, how much will each receive as a bonus?
Answer: _____

YOUR SCORE: _____ %

100%   YES—proceed to the next module
        NO —review this module or complete Appendix A.

_____

Note: if you had any errors on this posttest, analyze your areas of weakness.

Module 4: Ratio and Proportion

PRETEST

Instructions

1. Write the pretest without referring to any resource materials.

2. Correct the pretest using the answer guide.

3. If your score is 100 percent, proceed to the next module.

4. If you don't achieve 100 percent accuracy, read the learning package in this module and complete the exercises, concentrating on your weak areas as diagnosed by your pretest score.

Solve for N:

1. $3:N = 1:15$

2. $9:N = 3:4$

3. $\dfrac{N}{100} = \dfrac{5}{20}$

4. $\dfrac{25}{1} = \dfrac{100}{N}$

5. $\dfrac{8}{N} = \dfrac{12}{6}$

6. $\dfrac{1}{50} = \dfrac{N}{150}$

Express the following ratios as fractions, decimal numbers, and percents. Reduce fractions to lowest term.

Ratio	Fraction	Decimal	Percent
1:100	7.	8.	9.
1:5	10.	11.	12.
4:1 000	13.	14.	15.

Solve for N.

16. $\dfrac{0.25}{1} = \dfrac{0.125}{N}$

17. $\dfrac{2.2}{1} = \dfrac{N}{75}$

18. $\dfrac{1\,000}{1.5} = \dfrac{N}{3}$

19. $60:5 = 150:N$

20. You buy seven oranges and five apples. What is the ratio of oranges to apples?
Answer: _____

21. There are forty patients and eight staff members. What is the ratio of patients to staff? Express as a ratio in lowest terms.
Answer: _____

22. Your score is eighty-five percent on a math exam. What is the ratio of correct to incorrect answers? Express as a ratio in lowest terms.
Answer: _____

23. Your coffeemaker instructions state six scoops of coffee makes eight cups of coffee. How many scoops are needed to make two cups?
Answer: _____

24. Define the term *ratio*.

25. Define the term *proportion*.

YOUR SCORE: _____ %

100%   YES—proceed to the next module
         NO —complete this module

Note: if you had any errors on the pretest, analyze your areas of weakness.

Learning Package

> ### Objective
> **To solve for an unknown value using ratio and proportion; to express ratios as fractions, decimal numbers, and percents**

Definitions

Ratio: relationship that exists between two quantities. For example, a class of nursing students has 2 male and 148 female students. The ratio of males to females may be expressed as:

a to b   or   a:b

In this class the ratio of male to female is:

2 to 148   or   2:148

Stated in equivalent terms the ratio is 1:74

$$\left(\frac{2 \div 2}{148 \div 2} = \frac{1}{74} \right)$$

That is, for every 74 female students, there is 1 male student. (What do you think of this ratio? Your answer is probably influenced by your gender.)

In this sample, the ratio of male students to the total class would be expressed as follows:

male:total = 2:150   or   1:75

It is very important to be certain you are choosing the correct numbers for the ratio equation.

> Example: out of a basket of 200 apples, 57 are red and the remaining apples are green. The ratio of red to green is 57:143

Ratios are used commonly in everyday situations. When you are jogging, swimming, or cycling, perhaps you chart your performance in kilometres per hour or metres per minute. Walking at five kilometres per hour will burn up almost three calories per minute. Five kilometres per hour and three calories per minute are ratios.

Ratios are frequently used in drug calculations. The dosage strength of a medication can be expressed as a ratio.

> Example:
> 1 tablet contains 300 mg of drug. Ratio is 300 mg per tablet, or 300:1.

Exercise 4.1

Complete the following exercise without referring to the previous text. Correct using the answer guide.

You answered eighteen questions correctly on an exam with twenty questions.

1. What is the ratio of incorrect to correct answers?
Answer: _____

2. What is the ratio of correct to total answers?
Answer: _____

3. The drug bottle label states, "Each tablet contains 325 units." Express the ratio of this drug in units per tablet.
Answer: _____

4. A bottle of liquid medication states that each teaspoon contains 25 units. Express the ratio of units per teaspoon.
Answer: _____

5. In every hour of television programming that you watch, you also "enjoy" 12 minutes of advertising. Express the following as a ratio: time of advertising, in minutes, to time of actual program, in minutes.
Answer: _____

Expressing Ratios as Fractions, Decimal Numbers, and Percents

A ratio may be expressed as a fraction, a decimal number, or a percent. To convert a ratio to a fraction:

1. Place the first digit in the ratio over the second digit.

2. Simplify the fraction.

> Example: 2:50 as a fraction
>
> $$\frac{2}{50}$$
>
> Lowest term: $\frac{1}{25}$

To convert a ratio to a decimal number:

1. Express the ratio as a fraction.

2. Divide the numerator into the denominator.

3. Follow the rules for writing decimals.

> Example: 1:15 as a decimal
>
> Express as a fraction: $\frac{1}{15}$
>
> Divide: 1 divided by 15 = .066
> Follow rules for writing decimals: 0.066

To convert a ratio to a percent:

1. Express the ratio as a fraction.

2. Convert the fraction to a decimal number (divide numerator by denominator).

3. Multiply the decimal number by 100.

4. Add the percent sign.

Example: 1:20 as a percent

$$\frac{1}{20} = 0.05$$

$$0.05 \times 100 = 5$$

Answer: 5%

Similarly, a percent may be expressed as a ratio, since percent means "out of one hundred." To convert a percent to a ratio, place the percent over 100. Thus:

$$50\% = \frac{50}{100} = \frac{5}{10} = \frac{1}{2} = 1{:}2$$

$$0.5\% = \frac{0.5}{100} = \frac{5}{1\ 000} = \frac{1}{200} = 1{:}200$$

Exercise 4.2

Complete the following exercise without referring to the previous text. Correct using the answer guide.

Express the following ratios as fractions, decimal numbers, and percents. Express fractions in the lowest terms and round decimal numbers to the nearest tenth.

Ratio	Fraction	Decimal	Percent
2:50	1.	2.	3.
1:10	4.	5.	6.
7:9	7.	8.	9.
25:2	10.	11.	12.
50:1	13.	14.	15.
10:1	16.	17.	18.

Express these percents as ratios:

19. 75% =

20. 33.3% =

21. 50% =

22. 0.5% =

Proportion: expression of two equal or equivalent ratios. The two ratios are separated by an equal sign. For example; 2:3 = 4:6. In a true proportion, the product of the means equals the product of the extremes: thus,

$$
\begin{array}{c}
\overbrace{}^{\text{means}} \\
2{:}3 = 4{:}6 \\
\underbrace{}_{\text{extremes}} \\
2 \times 6 = 3 \times 4 \\
12 = 12
\end{array}
$$

Note: the **means** are the values in the **mi**ddle, the **extremes** are the values on the ends.

A proportion equation can be used to solve for an unknown quantity. The proportion equation is the simplest and most accurate approach to calculating drug dosages. In these situations, you have a known ratio; for example, the drug label states 325 mg per tablet or a ratio of 325:1. Another label states 100 mg in 2 mL or 100 mg:2 mL. The dosage that you wish to give is the unknown ratio. You know what strength to give but you must determine the volume to give (the number of tablets or millilitres, for example).

To solve for an unknown value (N) using proportion:

1. Write the known ratio first.

2. Write the unknown ratio.

3. Set up the proportion.

4. Multiply the means and the extremes; place the unknown value on the left.

5. Solve for the unknown. Recall that you must divide both sides of an equation by the same number.

6. Validate your answer. (Prove the answer.)

Example: 200:5 = 500:N

$200 \times N = 5 \times 500$

$200\,N = 2\,500$

$200\,N\,(\div 200) = 2\,500\,(\div 200)$

$N = 12.5$

Validation: $200 : 5 = 500 : 12.5$

$200 \times 12.5 = 5 \times 500$

$2\,500 = 2\,500$

Dosage calculations using proportion equations are illustrated in Module 7. Proceed to Exercise 4.3 to practice setting up true proportions.

Exercise 4.3

Complete the following exercise without referring to the previous text. Correct using the answer guide.

Solve for N:

1. 2:3 = N:12

2. 1:5 = N:125

3. 5:7 = 15:N

4. 25:1 = 50:N

5. 10:1 = 15:N

6. 75:2 = 50:N

7. 37:N = 100:1

8. 0.25:1 = 0.125:N

9. 250:1 000 = N:1

10. 10:1 000 = N:100

11. 1:8 = 1/2:N

12. 18:N = 5:300

13. 0.5:2 = N:4

14. 1/4:N = 6:12

15. N:6 = 1/100:1/10

For each of the following problems, show your work and validate the answer (show the proof).

16. To make six cups of coffee, you use four scoops of coffee and water. How many scoops do you need to make 24 cups?
Answer: _____

17. The pancake recipe requires 1 cup milk and 1 1/2 cups of mix. You have 4 cups of mix. How much milk should you add?
Answer: _____

18. You are making party bags for the birthday and want to put in 1 package of gum with 3 packages of mints. How many packages of gum do you need for 45 packages of mints?
Answer: _____

19. At the last hotdog day 22 children ate 33 hotdogs. How many hotdogs will you prepare for a class of 28 children?
Answer: _____

20. The fruit drink recipe calls for 1 cup of lime juice to 3 cups of apple juice. How much lime juice will you add to 20 cups of apple juice?
Answer: _____

POSTTEST

Instructions

1. Write the posttest without referring to any references.

2. Correct the posttest using the answer guide.

3. If your score is 100 percent, proceed to the next module.

4. If you don't achieve 100 percent accuracy, review the learning package in this module and rewrite the posttest. You may wish to seek further assistance through the additional exercises in Appendix B.

1. $3:7 = N:21$ $\hspace{8cm}$ N =

2. $\dfrac{N}{10} = \dfrac{4}{5}$ $\hspace{7cm}$ N =

3. $1:10 = N:100$ $\hspace{7cm}$ N =

4. Of sixty-two students in psychology, twenty-three are male. What is the ratio of male students to female students?
Answer: _____

5. A hockey player scores three goals in seventeen shots. What is the ratio of goals to shots?
Answer: _____

6. Define the term *ratio*.

7. Define the term *proportion*.

8. There are twenty-eight patients on a particular ward. The ratio of staff to patients is one to four. How many staff members are on this ward?
Answer: _____

9. Express the following statement as a ratio:

 Each teaspoon contains ten units of Drug A.

Answer: _____

10. Is the following relationship a proportion?

 6:32 = 24:100   Yes or No

11. Express 0.9% as a ratio.

Answer: _____

Express the following ratios as fractions, decimal numbers, and percents. Express fractions in lowest terms and round decimal numbers to the nearest tenth.

Ratio	Fraction	Decimal	Percent
1 : 1	12.	13.	14.
2 : 3	15.	16.	17.
1 : 1 000	18.	19.	20.

Express these ratios as fractions. Simplify if necessary.

21. 12:1 000

22. 16:500

23. 7:56

24. 26:65

Write the true proportion for each statement. Show the problem statement, the work to achieve the solution, and validation of the answer.

There are 12 red beads, and the pendant has 1 red bead for every 8 green beads. How many green beads are on the pendant?

25. Problem statement

26. Solution

27. Validation

The salt solution has 2 tablespoons of salt in 3 cups of water. How much salt is needed for 8 cups?

28. Problem statement

29. Solution

30. Validation

YOUR SCORE: _____ %

100%   YES—proceed to the next module
    NO —review this module or complete Appendix B.

Note: if you had any errors on the posttest, analyze your areas of weakness before reviewing.

Module 5: Systems of Measurement

PRETEST

Instructions

1. Write the pretest without referring to any resources.

2. Correct the pretest using the answer guide.

3. If your score is 100 percent, proceed to the next module.

4. If you don't achieve 100 percent accuracy, read the learning package in this module and complete the exercises, concentrating on your weak areas as diagnosed by your pretest score.

In the metric system, name the base units of:

	name	abbreviation
1. length		
2. weight (mass)		
3. substance		

Give the numerical value for each prefix:

4. deci _____

5. centi _____

6. milli _____

7. nano _____

8. micro _____

9. kilo _____

Do the following conversions of SI units:

10. 1 g = _____ mg

11. 1 L = _____ mL

12. 10 mg = _____ g

13. 1 kg = _____ g

14. 1 mg = _____ g

15. 250 mL = _____ L

16. 40 g = _____ kg

17. 200 mg = _____ g

18. 0.3 g = _____ mg

19. 1 m = _____ cm

20. 250 cm = _____ m

21. 0.6 g = _____ mg

Convert the following household measurements to SI units:

22. 2 fl oz. = _____ mL

24. 3 kg = _____ lb

23. 1 tsp = _____ mL

25. 6 ft = _____ cm

YOUR SCORE: _____ %

100%   YES—proceed to the next module
NO —review this module

Note: if you had any errors on the pretest, analyze your areas of weakness.

Learning Package

Objective
To convert between the base units and subunits of the SI system of measurement; to convert selected units of measurement from the SI system to other systems of measurement

---

Systems of Measurement

In the past, pharmacology has relied on several systems of measurement that have made dosage calculations quite confusing. This confusion has contributed to medication errors. Today the movement is towards standardization. All drugs should be ordered and dispensed in SI units. Drug orders should be written in units called *grams*, *milligrams*, and *millitres*. Nurses should not have to do conversions from one system of measurement to another, except for a few instances involving liquid medications, such as laxatives or antacids, or for instructions to the patient and family regarding uses of over-the-counter (OTC) drugs.

Note: if you are unfamiliar with any drug order written in nonstandardized units, consult with the prescribing physician or a pharmacist.

Three major systems of measurement have been used in pharmacology.

Household System

This system uses measures such as *drops*, *teaspoons*, and *tablespoons*. These measurements are most frequently used for prescription medications taken in the home and with such drugs as eye medications in the hospital. Figure 5.1 illustrates some household measures.

Apothecaries' System

This is a very old system whose basic units include *minims*, *ounces*, and *grains*. These measures have become almost obsolete except for some drug orders for laxatives, antacids, and cough syrups that may be written in ounces.* It's useful for you to be familiar with some of the units of these systems, since patients and families might be accustomed to these measures.† However, the official system of measurement in Canada is the SI system, and therefore emphasis is placed on this system in the module.

---

* Also some aspirin products, which are still labeled in grains.
† *Pounds* and *inches* are also part of this system.

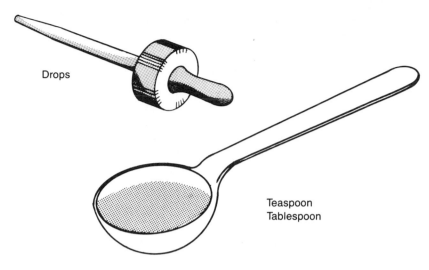

Figure 5.1   Household measures

SI System

The SI system, or Le Système International d'Unités, is essentially an expanded version of the metric system. It is a decimal system based on the number 10.

There are seven base units or building blocks in this system. The *base units* you will encounter most often in relation to medications are outlined in Table 5-A.

Table 5-A: Common Base Units

Name	Unit	Symbol
metre	unit of length	m
kilogram	unit of mass	kg
mole	unit of substance	mol

You are probably familiar with *metre* and *kilogram*. You've no doubt bought a metre of fabric or driven 100 kilometres. A metre is approximately the distance between the bottom of a door and its doorknob. Possibly you have bought a kilogram of meat. A kilogram is approximately equal in weight to a 1-litre carton of milk.

A *mole* is probably unfamiliar to you. It isn't a measurement of weight. A mole is an "amount of substance" defined as the number of atoms in exactly 12 g of the carbon-12 isotope. The number of entities in a mole of substance is 6.02×10^{23}. If your curiosity is aroused by this definition, you might appreciate further explanation. An anonymous and creative author described 1 mole of peas as follows:

> 10^{23} average-size peas would cover 250 planets the size of Earth with a blanket of peas 1 metre deep!

Obviously, 1 mole of peas occupies a much larger volume than a mole of potassium electrolytes.

Chemistry reports are expressed in molar units. This will become more significant to you when you read drug plasma levels reported in moles.

> Examples:
>
> insulin: 30 − 170 pmol/L
> (picomoles per litre)
>
> digoxin: < 2.6 nmol/L
> (nanomoles per litre)
>
> lithium: 0.6 − 1.2 mmol/L
> (millimoles per litre)

Note: laboratory values can vary slightly. Check the normal values written on the lab reports in your particular clinical setting.

In addition to these base units, one other measurement is not official SI but is of interest to health professionals. This is the unit of volume called the *litre*. For example, intravenous fluids are packaged in litre, 1 000 millilitre, containers.

Because the metre, kilogram, mole, and litre are relatively large units, the SI system uses prefixes to denote multiples and subunits. There are 16 prefixes, but only those used most frequently in relation to drug therapy are written in Table 5-B.

These numerical values are very important when converting base units and subunits of the SI system. You will do this frequently when administering medications and intravenous fluids to your patients. Mastering this module is an important step toward competence in calculating dosages.

Table 5-B: SI Subunits

Prefix	Symbol	Numerical Value
kilo	k	1 000
hecto	h	100
deci	d	0.1
centi	c	0.01
milli	m	0.001
micro	μ or mc	0.000 001
nano	n	0.000 000 001
pico	p	0.000 000 000 001

Note: the official symbol for *micro* is μ; however, some references use mc. Both abbreviations are acceptable.

Exercise 5.1

Review Table 5-B. Complete the following exercise without referring to the previous text. Correct using the answer guide.

Give the SI symbol for each of the following prefixes:

1. kilo

2. deci

3. centi

4. milli

5. micro

Write out the numerical value for each of the following prefixes:

6. kilo

7. nano

8. pico

9. milli

10. micro

11. centi

12. Name the 8 subunits of the SI system, as outlined in Table 5-B, from largest to smallest:

Rules for Writing SI Symbols

1. Symbols of units are written in lowercase initials, except when they are named after a person.

> Example:
> degree Celsius = C
> metre = m

2. Symbols are not pluralized. They are written without a period, except when the symbol occurs at the end of a sentence.

> Example:
> He weighs 10 kg.
> Ten kg is correct.

3. Decimals should be used instead of fractions.

> Example:
> $\frac{1}{2}$ is 0.5

4. Always place a zero before the decimal point when there is no whole number.

> Example:
> 0. 5 not .5

5. Just when you think you have this mastered . . . there's an exception to the rules. To avoid confusion with the number 1, write the word *litre* in full or use capital *L*. The capital *L* is also used with prefixes.

> Example:
> litre = L
> millilitre = mL

6. Writing numbers with more than three digits — that is, in the thousands — is slightly different from the traditional method. No comma is used. Instead a space is left, as shown in the example.

> Example:
> 1 000.039 78
> 23 000
> 217 860

7. Because old habits die slowly, there is one other point you should know. Although cc, *cubic centimetre*, isn't a standard SI unit, it's frequently used by health professionals — especially those of us who are BSI — before SI! The cc should be replaced by mL, millilitre; 1 cc is approximately equal to 1 mL.

Exercise 5.2

Complete the following exercise without referring to the previous text. Correct using the answer guide.

Indicate which of the following correctly adhere to the rules for writing SI symbols. Circle your choice.

1. metre = m or M

2. 10 kilograms = 10 kg or 10 kgs

3. $\frac{1}{2}$ millilitre = $\frac{1}{2}$ mL or 0.5 mL or 0.5 ml

4. litre = L or l

5. one thousand millilitres = 1 000 mL or 1,000 mL

6. Write fifty-one thousand, five hundred seventeen according to the SI rules.

7. True or false? 1 cc is approximately equal to 1 mL.

Converting SI Subunits to Base Units

The most common subunits encountered in drug therapy are *milli* and *micro*. In addition, you will frequently encounter *centi* in measurements of height or length. Table 5-C illustrates some relationships involving units of the SI system.

Table 5-C: Units and Values

Unit	Value
gram (g) to milligram (mg)	1 g = 1 000 mg
gram (g) to microgram (μg or mcg)	1 g = 1 000 000 μg (or mcg)
milligram (mg) to microgram (mg or mcg)	1 mg = 1 000 μg (or mcg)
litre (L) to millilitre (mL)	1 L = 1 000 mL
metre (m) to centimetre (cm)	1 m = 100 cm
metre (m) to millimetre (mm)	1 m = 1 000 mm

Conversion of subunits to base units and vice versa is a very simple exercise, involving multiplication or division by 10, 100, or 1 000. The trick, of course, is to remember whether to multiply or divide! The simplest approach is to use a proportion equation to solve. For example, how are grams converted to milligrams?

Example: 10 g = N mg
Known ratio is 1 g = 1 000 mg
Unknown ratio is 10 g = N mg

$$1 \text{ g}:1\ 000 \text{ mg} = 10 \text{ g}:N \text{ mg}$$
$$1 \text{ N} = 1\ 000 \times 10$$
$$N = 10\ 000$$
$$10 \text{ g} = 10\ 000 \text{ mg}$$

Validation:

$$1 \text{ g}:1\ 000 \text{ mg} = 10 \text{ g}:10\ 000 \text{ mg}$$
$$1 \times 10\ 000 = 1\ 000 \times 10$$
$$10\ 000 = 10\ 000$$

Remember to write the proportion with the known ratio on the left, the unknown ratio on the right. Be sure that each side of the equation is set up in the same way. In the previous example, the known ratio is stated as g:mg, so the unknown ratio must also be stated as g:mg. Examine the following problem and determine the various ways that the proportion could be stated.

How many milligrams are there in 0.2 g?

Write your answers before verifying. There are at least three ways to state a proportion equation to solve this question.

The answers are:

    a. 1 g:1 000 mg = 0.2 g:N mg

    b. 1 g:0.2 g = 1 000 mg:N mg

    c. 1 000 mg:1 g = N mg:0.2 g

Solutions for each equation show that the proportion equations all yield the same answer.

    a. 1 g:1 000 mg = 0.2 g:N mg

$$1 N = 1 000 \times 0.2$$
$$N = 200$$

  Answer is 200 mg

  Validation: 1 g:1 000 mg = 0.2 g:200 mg

$$1 \times 200 = 1 000 \times 0.2$$
$$200 = 200$$

    b. 1 g:0.2 g = 1 000 mg:N mg

$$1 N = 0.2 \times 1 000$$
$$N = 200$$

  Answer is 200 mg

  Validation: 1 g:0.2 g = 1 000 mg:200 mg

$$1 \times 200 = 0.2 \times 1 000$$
$$200 = 200$$

    c. 1 000 mg:1 g = N mg:0.2 g

$$1 N = 1 000 \times 0.2$$
$$N = 200$$

  Answer is 200 mg

  Validation: 1 000 mg:1 g = 200 mg: 0.2 g

$$1 000 \times 0.2 = 1 \times 200$$
$$200 = 200$$

Exercise 5.3

Complete the following exercise without referring to the previous text. Correct using the answer guide.

1. 1 L =   _____ mL

2. 1 kg =   _____ g

3. 1 m =   _____ cm

4. 1 cc =   _____ mL

5. 1 g =   _____ μg

6. 250 mL =   _____ L

7. 0.5 g =   _____ mg

8. 2 m =   _____ cm

9. 1 mg =   _____ μg

10. 1 000 μg = _____ g

11. 300 mg = _____ g

12. 800 g = _____ kg

13. 150 cm _____ m

14. 0.75 g = _____ mg

15. 2 500 g = _____ kg

Common Conversions

Because of the common usage of inches, pounds, and fluid ounces by the public and professionals, it is practical to know the following conversions from the SI system to the household and apothecaries' systems. Table 5-D lists these common conversions.

Table 5-D: Common Conversions

Unit	SI	Household/ Apothecaries
weight	kg	pounds
	1 kg =	2.2 pounds (lbs)
height	cm	inches
	2.54 cm =	1 inch (in)
volume	mL	teaspoon
	4 to 5 mL =	1 teaspoon (tsp)
	mL	fluid ounces
	30 mL =	1 ounce (oz)
	480 mL	1 pint = 16 oz

Example: how do you convert 2 kg to its equivalent in lbs?

$$1\,kg{:}2.2\,lbs = 2\,kg{:}N\,lbs$$
$$N = 2.2 \times 2$$
$$N = 4.4$$

Answer is 4.4 lbs

$$88\,lbs = ?\,kg$$
$$1\,kg{:}2.2\,lbs = N\,kg{:}88\,lbs$$
$$2.2\,N = 88$$
$$2.2\,N\,(\div 2.2) = 88\,(\div 2.2)$$
$$N = 40$$

Answer is 40 kg

$$3\,oz = ?\,mL$$
$$1\,oz{:}30\,mL = 3\,oz{:}N\,mL$$
$$N = 30 \times 3$$
$$N = 90$$

Answer is 90 mL

Exercise 5.4

Review Table 5-D and master the conversions before completing the following exercise. Answer the questions without referring back to Table 5-D. Correct using the answer guide.

You are admitting Mr. Jones, who cannot be weighed. He tells you that his weight is 175 lb.

1. Convert this to kg.

2. Round to the nearest tenth.

3. Round to the nearest kg.

Tim's height is 140 cm.

4. Express Tim's height in inches.

5. Express Tim's height in feet and inches.

6. The label states, "For ages 2 to 3, give 1 tsp." Convert this measurement to mL.

7. The order is: Magnolax 1 oz. Convert to mL.

POSTTEST

Instructions

1. Write the posttest without referring to any reference materials.

2. Correct the posttest using the answer guide.

3. If your score is 100 percent, proceed to the next module.

4. If you don't achieve 100 percent, review the appropriate sections of the learning package in this module and rewrite the posttest.

1. 2 L = —————— mL

2. 250 mg = —————— g

3. 2 000 mg = ————— g

4. 6 g = —————— mg

5. 7 kg = —————— g

6. 5 000 mL = ————— L

7. 1.25 mg = —————— g

8. 0.003 g = —————— mg

9. 2.5 g = —————— mg

10. 0.5 L = —————— mL

11. 1 456 g = —————— kg

12. 0.5 mg = —————— g

13. 1 mg —————— μg

14. 1.7 m = —————— cm

15. 179 cm = —————— m

16. 0.5 g = —————— mg

17. 250 mL = —————— L

18. 1.34 g = —————— mg

19. 10 g = —————— μg

20. 79 kg = —————— mg

Give the numerical value for each prefix:

21. centi

22. milli

23. micro

24. kilo

25. deci

Module 6: Medication Orders and Dosage Forms

PRETEST

Instructions

1. Write the pretest without referring to any resources.

2. Correct the pretest using the answer guide.

3. If your score is 100 percent, proceed to the next module.

4. If you don't achieve 100 percent accuracy, read the learning package in this module and complete the exercises, concentrating on your weak areas as diagnosed by your pretest score.

Interpret each of the following medication orders and write out the underlined abbreviation in full:

1. Morphine sulfate 10–15 mg I.M. q.4h. p.r.n.

2. Insulin 6 units S.C. stat.

3. Metoclopramide (Reglan) 10 mg P.O. a.c. t.i.d.

4. Aluminum hydroxide 30 mL P.O. 1 h p.c. t.i.d.

5. Flurazepam hydrochloride (Dalmane) 15 mg P.O. h.s.

Refer to Figure 6.1 and answer questions 6 to 9.

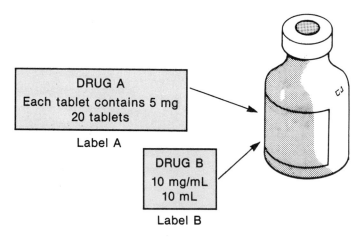

DRUG A
Each tablet contains 5 mg
20 tablets

Label A

DRUG B
10 mg/mL
10 mL

Label B

Figure 6.1 Drug labels A and B

	Label	
	A	B
form of the drug	6.	7.
dosage strength	8.	9.

List the parts of a medication order. All medication orders should include the patient name, the drug name, the frequency or time of administration, and the

10. d _____ ,

11. and r _____ .

12. A single-dose ampule labeled 25 mg/mL contains exactly 1 mL of liquid. True or false?

Match the abbreviation in column 1 with the correct expression in column 2.

Column 1	Column 2
13. _____ p.c.	A. twice daily
14. _____ stat.	B. capsule
15. _____ elix.	C. ointment
16. _____ ung.	D. at bedtime
17. _____ tab.	E. after meals
18. _____ a.c.	F. elixir
19. _____ cap.	G. immediately
20. _____ b.i.d.	H. tablet
21. _____ h.s.	I. before meals
22. _____ S.C.	J. subcutaneous

Read the label below and answer questions 23 to 30.

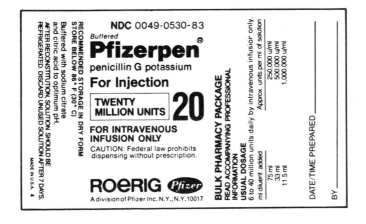

23. State the three options for volume of diluent that may be added to the vial.

24. What is the total amount of drug contained in this vial?

25. If 33 mL of diluent is added, what is the strength of the solution?

26. State the generic name of the drug.

27. State the trade name of the drug.

28. State the route of administration for this drug.

29. State the usual daily dosage range.

30. The solution is reconstituted on the fifteenth day of the month. When should unused solution be discarded?

Define each of the following terms in your own words and according to the module definitions:

31. solute

32. solution

33. solvent

34. strength or concentration

YOUR SCORE: _____ %

100%   YES—proceed to the next module
         NO —complete this module

Note: if you had any errors on the pretest, analyze your areas of weakness.

Learning Package

```
                        Objective
To interpret medication orders;
to determine concentrations of
liquid medications and describe
the reconstitution of powdered
drugs
```

Medication Orders

In most clinical settings, medications are prescribed by a physician, dispensed by a pharmacist, and administered by a nurse. All medication orders should include the patient's name, the drug, dose, route, and frequency or time of administration.

```
Example: morphine sulfate 10 mg I.M.          stat
         drug              dose  route   time or frequency
```

Obviously this order would also specify the recipient!

Note: dose and dosage both refer to the exact amount of medicine to be given or taken at a specified time.

Commonly Used Abbreviations

The first step is correct interpretation of the medication order. Handwriting jokes aside, even a legible order is usually written in shorthand. It's important to learn this "new language." Abbreviations vary considerably among institutions and prescribers. Some are easily misinterpreted and can lead to error. For example, q.d., o.d., and OD have all been used to mean "daily" or "once a day." However, OD also means "right eye." The abbreviation, q.d., can also be confused with q.i.d., which would result in a very serious error. For example, digoxin (Lanoxin) would be given four times a day instead of only once. The letter "u" for units can be easily misread as a 0. For example, serious drug errors have occurred because 6 u of insulin was read as 60. The abbreviations listed in Box 6-A have become widely accepted. Some have been used in the calculation problems in this workbook. You are urged to verify acceptable abbreviations used in the practice setting.

Box 6-A: Commonly Used Abbreviations

a.c.	before meals ($\frac{1}{2}$ hour before meals)
b.i.d.	twice daily
cap.	capsule
elix.	elixir
ext.	extract
h.s.	at bedtime
I.M. or i.m.	intramuscular
I.V. or i.v.	intravenous
mEq.	milliequivalent
p.c.	after meals ($\frac{1}{2}$ hour after meals)
P.O. or p.o.	by mouth
p.r.n.	as necessary (according to necessity)
q.h.	every hour
q.4h.	every 4 hours
q.i.d.	4 times a day
q.s.	as much as required
S.C. or s.c.	subcutaneous
stat.	immediately
tab.	tablet
t.i.d.	3 times a day
u.	unit
ung.	ointment

Note: sometimes these abbreviations are written without periods; for example, bid, po.
Unit: a drug measure based on a specific effect; for example, a unit of insulin is a standardized amount that lowers blood sugar.
Milliequivalent: measurement of combining power rather than weight.

Exercise 6.1

Complete the following exercise without referring to the previous text. Correct using the answer guide.

Interpret the following medication orders. Write out each of the underlined abbreviations in full.

1. Meperidine (Demerol) 50–75 mg I.M. q.3-4h. p.r.n.

2. Acetaminophen (Tylenol) 650 mg P.O. q.4h.

3. Codeine sulfate 60 mg P.O. stat and q.4h.

4. Penicillin 500 000 units I.V. q.i.d.

5. Phenobarbital elix. 100 mg h.s.

List the Parts of a Medication Order:

6.   7.

8.   9.

10.

Medication Labels

The medication label contains very important information. Some labels are clearly presented, provided your vision is satisfactory! Other labels are confusing. They aren't standardized as to what information is included or how it is presented. It's important to develop the habit of thoroughly studying the information and instructions on drug labels. Accompanying literature also provides useful information. Check your habits: the last time you bought a piece of equipment — tape recorder, video machine, or pocket calculator — *did you read the instructions*?

The label below illustrates the type of information that should be included in drug packaging.

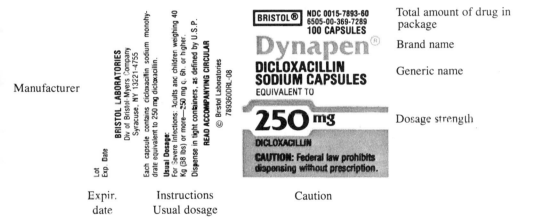

Manufacturer

Expir.   Instructions   Caution
date   Usual dosage

Total amount of drug in package

Brand name

Generic name

Dosage strength

Exercise 6.2

Complete the following exercise without referring to the previous text. Correct using the answer guide.

Refer to the label below and answer questions 1 to 3.

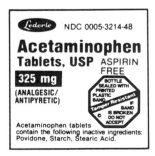

1. State the form of the drug.

2. What is the dosage strength?

3. State the drug name.

Refer to the label below and answer questions 4 to 10.

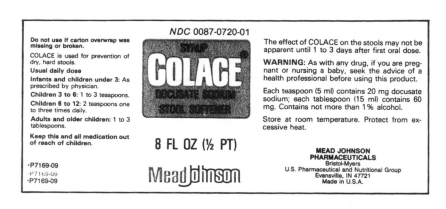

NDC 0087-0720-01

Do not use if carton overwrap was missing or broken.

COLACE is used for prevention of dry, hard stools.

Usual daily dose

Infants and children under 3: As prescribed by physician.

Children 3 to 6: 1 to 3 teaspoons.

Children 6 to 12: 2 teaspoons one to three times daily.

Adults and older children: 1 to 3 tablespoons.

Keep this and all medication out of reach of children.

·P7169-09
·P7169-09
·P7169-09

COLACE

DOCUSATE SODIUM
STOOL SOFTENER

8 FL OZ (½ PT)

Mead Johnson

The effect of COLACE on the stools may not be apparent until 1 to 3 days after first oral dose.

WARNING: As with any drug, if you are pregnant or nursing a baby, seek the advice of a health professional before using this product.

Each teaspoon (5 ml) contains 20 mg docusate sodium; each tablespoon (15 ml) contains 60 mg. Contains not more than 1% alcohol.

Store at room temperature. Protect from excessive heat.

MEAD JOHNSON
PHARMACEUTICALS
Bristol-Myers
U.S. Pharmaceutical and Nutritional Group
Evansville, IN 47721
Made in U.S.A.

4. State the trade name of the drug.

5. State the generic name of the drug.

6. State the usual dose for adults. Convert the dose to mL.

7. What is the form of the drug?

8. What is the dosage strength of the drug?

9. What is the total volume contained in this bottle (in mL)?

10. If an adult took 2 tsp daily, how many days would the drug in this bottle last?

Packaging of Medications

Medications are prepared and packaged in a variety of forms. Oral doses are provided in compressed tablets, capsules, and liquids. Some tablets are scored and can be easily broken in half. Injectables are packaged in both single-dose and multiple-dose containers.

An important point should be made about the single-dose ampule. The ampule may state that N mg per mL are contained premixed for a single dose. However, the ampule contains slightly more than 1 mL, to allow for some loss of solution within the needle and syringe. Therefore, always carefully calculate and measure the correct dose, and do not draw up the entire contents of an ampule. A similar point can be made regarding vials and bags of intravenous fluids. All packages of liquid medication contain extra fluid.

Injectables are prepared as liquids ready for injection or in powdered form requiring reconstitution with a diluent. The procedure for reconstitution and calculation of these products is described in Module 7.

Many drugs are prepared in liquid form. The following discussion briefly reviews terminology associated with solutions.

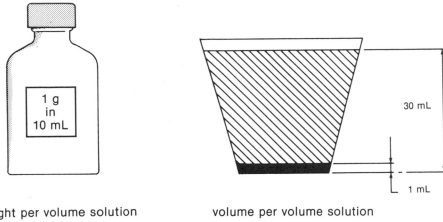

weight per volume solution   volume per volume solution

Figure 6.2   Types of solutions

Types of Solutions

Definitions

A **solution** is a homogeneous mixture that contains one or more dissolved substances in a liquid. For example, when you add sugar to your tea you are creating a solution.

A **solvent** is the liquid in which another substance is dissolved. In the above example, the tea is the solvent.

A **solute** is the substance dissolved in the solvent. In our example, sugar is a solute.

Some drugs are available in solution; the drug is the solute, and water is usually the solvent. In other instances, solvents used include normal saline, alcohol, or other liquids.

When drugs are prepared in solution, they are described by the **strength** or **concentration** of the solution. The strength or concentration of a solution is determined by the amount of solute dissolved in a given amount of solvent. For example, did you put 1 tsp or 2 tsp of sugar in your cup of tea?

An example of strength of solutions is demonstrated by the preparation of heparin. This is done in varying strengths, such as 1 000 units per mL and 10 000 units per mL. The latter preparation is 10 times greater in concentration than the former.

There are many types of solutions and, in most instances involving drugs, they are premixed. The two types of solutions that are relevant in medication therapy are illustrated in Figure 6.2, then explained further.

A **weight per volume** solution: the solute is weighed, but the solvent is expressed in volume: g to mL. This is the most common type of medication solution.

Most intravenous solutions are expressed as a weight per volume type of solution: a given weight of dextrose, in g, is dissolved in a certain volume of water, in mL.

A **volume per volume** solution: both the solute and the solvent are measured in the same units of volume. For example, 1 mL of drug may be dissolved in 10 mL of water or alcohol.

The label indicates whether the solution is a weight per volume (w/v) or volume per volume (v/v) type of solution by giving the units of measurement of the solute and the solvent.

> 1 tsp in 1 fluid oz is a volume per volume
> 1 g per 100 mL is a weight per volume

Medication labels indicate the strength of the drug available in solution. The strength may be stated as a percentage or as a ratio. For example, a 5% solution has 5 g of medication in every 100 mL of solution. If the label states 1:1 000, this means that 1 g of drug is dissolved in 1 000 mL (or that the strength is 1 mg per mL). The amount of drug dissolved in solution may also be stated using other units of measure: examples include mmol, mEq, and u.

Exercise 6.3

Complete the following exercise without referring to the previous text. Correct using the answer guide.

Complete each of the following sentences with the most appropriate term.

1. A homogeneous mixture that contains one or more dissolved substances in a liquid is called a _____.

2. The substance that is dissolved in a solution is called a _____.

3. In a solution, the liquid in which a substance is dissolved is called a _____.

Read the description of this drug, then answer questions 4 and 5.

> Add 4.6 mL of sterile water to obtain
> penicillin G potassium 200 000 units per mL.

4. In this drug solution, name the solute.

5. In this drug solution, name the solvent.

Indicate whether the following sentence is true or false:

6. The strength or concentration of a solution is determined by the amount of solute dissolved in a given amount of solvent.

For the following questions, choose the best answer.

7. Which solution has the greater concentration?
   a. 1 000 units per 1 mL
   b. 10 000 units per 1 mL

8. The labels on two vials of the same medication indicate that the concentrations are:

   Drug A: 10 mg/mL
   Drug B: 100 mg in 10 mL

   Is the concentration of Drug A:
   a. the same as that of Drug B?
   b. less than that of Drug B?
   c. greater than that of Drug B?

Complete questions 9 to 12 by indicating the unit of measurement for the solute and the solvent for each type of solution. Choose your response from this list of units: g, mg, mL.

9. In a weight per volume solution, the unit of measurement of the solute is a _____.

10. In a weight per volume solution, the unit of measurement of the solvent is a _____.

11. In a volume per volume solution, the unit of measurement of the solute is a _____.

12. In a volume per volume solution, the unit of measurement of the solvent is a _____.

Indicate whether the following solutions are weight per volume or volume per volume type:

13. A solution that has 5 g of solute, pure drug, dissolved in 100 mL of solvent is termed a _____ solution.

14. You have mixed 5 mL of lemon juice with 250 mL of water. You have prepared a _____ type of solution.

POSTTEST

Instructions

1. Write the posttest without referring to any reference materials.

2. Correct the posttest using the answer guide.

3. If your score is 100 percent, proceed to the next module.

4. If you don't achieve 100 percent, review the learning package in this module and rewrite the posttest.

Part One

Complete the crossword in Figure 6.3 with the correct abbreviation. (Value: 16)

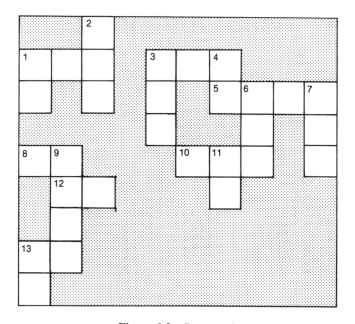

Figure 6.3 Crossword

Across

1. as required
3. every 4 hours
5. immediately
8. after meals
10. twice daily
12. before meals
13. as much as is required

Down

1. by mouth
2. ointment
3. four times a day
4. at bedtime
6. three times a day
7. tablet
9. capsules
11. intramuscular
13. every hour

Part Two

Read the label on p. 89 and answer questions 1 to 8.

1. What is the form of the drug?

2. What is the volume in each vial?

3. What is the concentration of the drug?

4. How many vials does the box contain?

5. What storage instructions should you follow?

6. The order on the chart states: morphine 10 mg I.M. q.3h. p.r.n. Is this drug form appropriate for this route of administration?

7. How often can the patient receive the morphine (for the order in question 6)?

8. You are preparing the dosage (question 6) and notice slight discoloration. What instructions should you follow?

Interpret the following orders. Do not use any abbreviations.

9. Digoxin 250 mcg P.O. daily

10. Indocid 50 mg P.O. t.i.d.

11. Phenobarbital 25 mg P.O. h.s.

12. Benadryl 25 mg P.O. q.i.d.

13. Pro-Banthine 15 mg P.O. a.c. and 30 mg h.s.

14. Demerol 75 mg I.M. q.3-4h. p.r.n.

15. Amikacin 15 mg/kg/day I.V.

Define each of the following terms in your own words and according to the module definitions.

16. solute

17. solution

18. solvent

19. strength or concentration

20. The term *percent concentration* describes the strength of a solution by stating the parts of solute, or pure drug, in how many parts of solution?

YOUR SCORE: _____ %

100%   YES—proceed to the next module
           NO —review this module

Note: if you had any errors on the posttest, analyze your areas of weakness.

Module 7: Dosage Calculations of Oral Medications

PRETEST

Instructions

1. Write the pretest without referring to any resources.

52. Correct the pretest using the answer guide.

3. If your score is 100 percent, proceed to the next module.

4. If you do not achieve 100 percent accuracy, read the learning package in this module and complete the exercises, concentrating on your weak areas as diagnosed by your pretest score.

Calculate the following dosages.

Note: be careful to include the appropriate unit of measure with your answer, for example, tablet, mg, mL. Round decimal numbers to the nearest tenth.

1. The order is: 0.015 g of Drug X. The tablets are 5 mg each. Determine the correct dose in tablets.

2. From aspirin tablets of 325 mg each, determine the correct dose in tablets for 650 mg P.O.

3. The order is: cephalexin (Keflex) 1 g P.O. q.6h. The label indicates that the bottle contains 500-mg tabs. Determine the correct dose in tablets.

4. The patient is to receive theophylline (Theo-Dur) 450 mg P.O. p.c. The bottle contains 300-mg tabs. Determine the correct dosage in tablets.

5. The order is: bromocriptine mesylate (Parlodel) 5 mg P.O. daily. The available dose is 2.5-mg tabs. Determine the correct dosage in tablets.

6. The order is: nadolol (Corgard) 40 mg P.O. h.s. The bottle is labeled: ''nadolol 80-mg tabs.'' Determine the correct dosage in tablets.

7. The patient is to receive levothyroxine sodium (Synthroid) 0.15 mg P.O. once daily. The bottle label reads: Synthroid 0.05 mg/tab. Determine the correct dosage in tablets.

8. The order is: digoxin (Lanoxin) 0.125 mg P.O. q.a.m. The bottle is labeled: digoxin 0.25-mg tabs. Determine the correct dosage in tablets.

9. The order is: cloxacillin sodium (Orbenin) 500 mg q.i.d. × 3 weeks. The available dosage is 250-mg capsules. How many capsules will be required for a 3-week supply?

Refer to the drug labels below and answer questions 10 to 20.

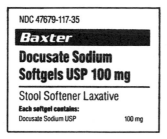

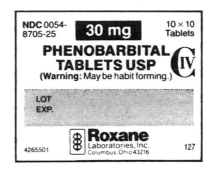

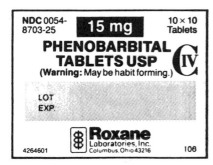

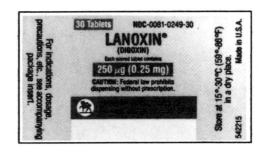

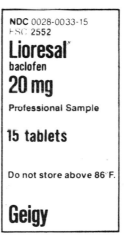

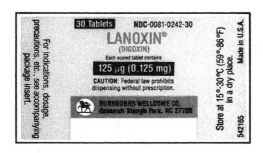

For each of the following drug orders, state the correct amount to administer. Be sure to state the dosage strength of the drug; for example, give 2 tablets of 10 mg dosage strength.

10. Digoxin 125 mcg P.O. daily

11. Phenobarbital 15 mg P.O. b.i.d.

12. Baclofen 10 mg P.O. t.i.d. × 3 days

13. Docusate sodium 200 mg h.s.

14. Phenobarbital 15 mg P.O. in a.m. and 30 mg P.O. h.s.

15. Lanoxin 0.25 mg P.O. daily

16. A woman accidentally took 2 tablets of her digoxin (0.125 mg). How many mcg did she ingest?

17. Phenobarbital 45 mg P.O. b.i.d.

18. Baclofen 5 mg t.i.d. for 4 days, then 10 mg t.i.d. × 3 days. Calculate each dose, then state how many tablets are required for the 7 days.

19. A child swallowed all of the 20-mg Lioresal tablets. What was the total dose ingested?

20. The order states: phenobarbital 30 mg P.O. b.i.d. and 45 mg h.s. Calculate each of the doses and state the total daily dose given.

YOUR SCORE: _____ %

100%   YES—proceed to the next module
         NO —complete this module

Note: if you had any errors on the pretest, analyze your areas of weakness.

Learning Package

```
┌─────────────────────────────────┐
│           Objective             │
│ To calculate dosages of oral    │
│ and parenteral medications      │
│ accurately                      │
└─────────────────────────────────┘
```

The previous modules presented a review of basic arithmetic skills: addition, subtraction, multiplication, and division of whole numbers, decimal numbers, and fractions. These skills are required for accurate dosage calculations.

Note: the terms *dose* and *dosage* can be used interchangeably. Each term means the amount of medication to be given.

Frequently, nurses must calculate and administer drugs or instruct patients and families in calculations for self-medication. Accurate dosage calculation is extremely important to patient safety. This module describes how to calculate oral medications and provides several practice exercises to develop your skill.

Calculating Dosages of Tablets

The oral route is the most common means of drug administration. Use ratio and proportion to calculate the number of tablets or capsules.

Example:

The order is for diazepam (Valium) 5 mg P.O. The bottle is labeled: diazepam 10-mg tablets.

Known ratio: 10 mg/1 tab
Unknown ratio: 5 mg/N tab

Solve: $10 \text{ mg} : 1 \text{ tab} = 5 \text{ mg} : N \text{ tab}$

$$10 N = 5$$

$$N = \frac{5}{10} = 0.5$$

Answer: give $\frac{1}{2}$ tab

Validation: $10:1 = 5:0.5$

Note: always check your answer "intuitively." Does it make sense? In the previous example, 5 mg was ordered. This is *less* than the amount available. This answer does make sense.

Sometimes the dose ordered and the dose on hand are in the same unit of measure.

Example:

The physician orders ascorbic acid 100 mg P.O. The dose on hand is in 50-mg tabs.

Known ratio: 50 mg/1 tab
Unknown ratio: 100 mg/N tab
Solve using proportion equation.

$$50{:}1 = 100{:}N$$
$$50\,N = 100$$
$$N = \frac{100}{50} = 2$$

Answer: give 2 tabs
Validation: $50{:}1 = 100{:}2$

In other situations, the dose ordered and the dose on hand are in different units.

Example:

The order is for 1.5 g of sulfisoxazole (Gantrisin). Available: 500-mg tabs.

Note: The dose ordered and the dose on hand must be written in the same units.

Step 1: convert the order to the same unit as the dose on hand. (Review Module 5 if necessary.)

1.5 g = ? mg
     = 1 500 mg

Step 2: solve using proportion equation.
Known ratio: 500 mg/1 tab
Unknown ratio: 1 500 mg/N tab

$$\text{Solve: } 500{:}1 = 1\ 500{:}N$$
$$500\,N = 1\ 500$$
$$N = \frac{1\ 500}{500} = 3$$

Answer: give 3 tabs
Validation: $500{:}1 = 1\ 500{:}3$

Exercise 7.1

Complete the following exercise without referring to the previous text. Correct using the answer guide. Be *careful* to state your answer in full: include tablets, capsules, or other pill forms in your response.

1. On hand are sulfisoxazole (Gantrisin) tablets of 500 mg each. How many tablets are required for a single dose of 1 g?

2. The order is: sulfisoxazole (Gantrisin) 1.5 g P.O. t.i.d. The available strength is 500-mg tablets. Determine the correct amount to administer.

3. The order is: caffeine 0.2 g p.r.n. The tablets are labeled 100 mg each. Determine the correct amount to administer.

4. You are to give meperidine (Demerol) 75 mg P.O. for pain. The scored tablets on hand are 50 mg each. Determine the correct amount to administer.

5. The order is: hydrochlorothiazide (HydroDIURIL) 100 mg P.O. daily. The available tablets are labeled 50 mg each. Determine the correct amount to administer.

6. The patient is to receive 30 mg P.O. of Drug A. There are two dosage strengths available. One bottle is labeled 5-mg tablets; another bottle contains 20-mg tablets. Determine the correct amount to administer. Be certain to indicate which tablet strength you are using.

7. The order is: digoxin (Lanoxin) 0.125 mg P.O. daily. The available scored tablets are 0.25-mg strength. Determine the correct amount to administer.

8. The order is: levothyroxine sodium (Eltroxin) 0.1 mg P.O. daily. The tablets are labeled 0.05 mg each. Determine the correct amount to administer.

9. The patient is to receive 0.05 mg of Drug B. The scored tablets are labeled 0.1 mg each. Determine the correct amount to administer.

10. The order is for 0.5 g of an antibiotic. The bottle is labeled 250-mg capsules. Determine the correct amount to administer.

Calculating Dosages of Liquids

Many medications are administered orally in suspensions and parenterally in solutions. Consider the following situation:

> Example:
>
> The order is thioridazine hydrochloride (Mellaril) 60 mg P.O. p.r.n.
> On hand is Mellaril 25 mg/5 mL. What amount should be administered?

Obviously the answer must be expressed in volume. How many mL should the patient receive?

Solve this problem using ratio and proportion. Once again you have a known ratio and an unknown ratio.

> Known ratio: 25 mg/5 mL
> Unknown ratio: 60 mg/N mL
> 25 mg:5 mL = 60 mg:N mL
>
> $25 N = 60 \times 5$
> $N = 300/25$
> $N = 12$
>
> Answer is 12 mL
> Validation: 25:5 = 60:12

Check that each side of the equation expresses the same relationship; that is, mg to mL.

Dosage errors often result from carelessness. Whenever you calculate a dosage, check the answer to see if it seems reasonable. For example, in this problem would an answer of 1 mL seem reasonable?

Note: be certain to express the units of weight and volume in your ratio. It is easy to come up with an answer and then be left wondering — N = 10 (but 10 *what*? mg? mL?).

Place "12" in the original equation, and you know that the answer is 12 mL.

The labels below and on the facing page illustrate several drugs prepared in liquid form for oral administration. Read the labels carefully, noting that some liquids are "suspension," and others are solutions or elixirs. Review these definitions and proceed to Exercise 7.2.

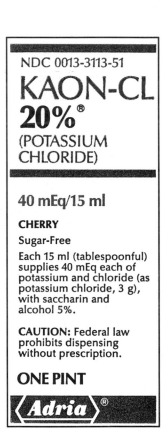

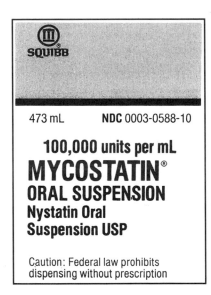

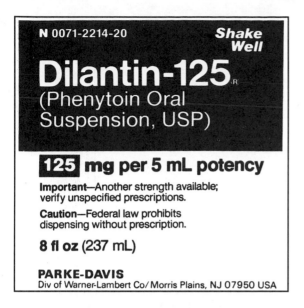

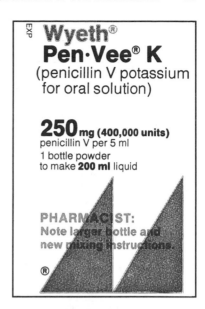

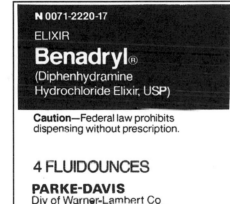

Elixir P-D 2220 for prescription dispensing only.

Contains—12.5 mg diphenhydramine hydrochloride in each 5 mL. Alcohol, 14%.

Dose—Adults, 2 to 4 teaspoonfuls; children over 20 lb, 1 to 2 teaspoonfuls; three or four times daily.

See package insert.

Keep this and all drugs out of the reach of children.

Store below 30°C (86°F). Protect from freezing and light.

Exp date and lot

2220G I02

Solution: one or more drugs are dissolved in water.

Suspension: fine particles of a drug are suspended in a liquid base; appears cloudy; shake well before administering; includes emulsions, magmas, and gels.

Elixirs: aromatic, sweetened solutions containing a dissolved medication; contain various percentages of alcohol. Determine the alcohol content of the Kaon-Cl and the Benadryl from the labels above and on the facing page.

Exercise 7.2

Complete the exercise without referring to the previous text. If you have difficulty doing conversions between the household and metric systems, review Table 5-D. Correct using the answer guide.

Refer to the labels above and answer questions 1 to 20.

State the total volume, in mL, in each drug container.

1. Mycostatin oral suspenion   _____ mL

2. Pen-Vee K oral solution   _____ mL

3. Kaon-Cl   _____ mL

4. Benadryl elixir   _____ mL

5. Dilantin suspension   _____ mL

For each order state the volume to be administered.

6. Benadryl 12.5 mg. How many mL?

7. Benadryl 12.5 mg. How many tsp?

8. Benadryl 25 mg. How many mL?

9. Dilantin 100 mg. How many mL?

10. Phenytoin 125 mg. How many tsp?

11. Potassium chloride 20 mEq. How many mL?

12. Pen-Vee K 200 000 units. How many mL?

13. Pen-Vee K 200 mg. How many mL?

14. Pen-Vee K 400 000 units. How many tsp?

15. Mycostatin 100 000 units. How many mL?

For each of the following orders, calculate the total number of doses that can be given from the volume indicated on the drug label.

16. Dilantin 125 mg P.O. t.i.d.

17. Benadryl 50 mg P.O. b.i.d.

18. Penicillin V Potassium 400 000 units P.O. t.i.d.

19. Nystatin oral suspension 100 000 q.i.d. dropped into mouth and held before swallowing.

20. Potassium chloride 20 mEq P.O. daily.

POSTTEST

Instructions

1. Write the posttest without referring to any reference materials.

2. Correct the posttest using the answer guide.

3. If your score is 100 percent, proceed to the next module.

4. If you don't achieve 100 percent, complete Appendix C or review the appropriate sections of the learning package in this module and rewrite the posttest.

5. Be careful to include units with all answers (e.g., mg, mL, tabs). Round decimal numbers to the nearest tenth.

1. The order is: phenobarbital (Luminal) 0.3 g P.O. The dose on hand is in 100-mg tabs. How many tablets should you give?

2. The order is: probenecid (Benemid) 750 mg P.O. The dose on hand is 500-mg (scored) tabs. Determine the correct dosage to administer.

3. From reserpine (Serpasil) tablets of 0.25 mg each, determine the correct dosage for an order of 0.5 mg P.O.

4. Aspirin 0.65 g is ordered. You have tablets of 325 mg each. How many tablets should you give?

5. The patient is to receive 0.8 mg of drug S. The drug is labeled 0.4 mg/tab. How many tablets should be given?

6. The physician orders 0.125 mg of digoxin (Lanoxin) P.O. daily. The drug is labeled 125 mcg/tab. How many tablets would the patient require for a 2-week supply?

7. You are to give 2 000 mg of Drug B. The label indicates that each tablet is 1 g. How many tablets should you give?

8. The physician orders 75-mg tabs p.r.n. for pain. The dose on hand is 50 mg scored tabs. How many tablets would you give?

9. The patient is to receive elixir of phenobarbital 4 mg. The bottle in the drug cabinet reads 4 mg/5 mL. How many mL should be administered?

10. The order is for streptomycin 500 mg q.6h. The drug label reads 5 g/12.5 mL. How many mL should the patient receive?

Refer to the labels below and answer questions 11 to 20. Round decimal numbers to the nearest tenth.

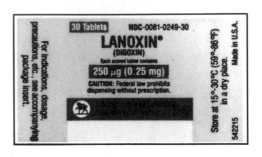

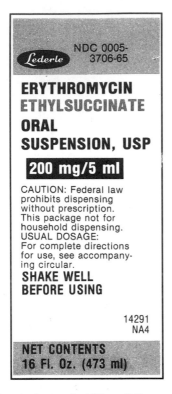

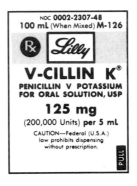

11. Give erythromycin 150 mg P.O.

12. A mother gave her child 1 tsp of erythromycin. What dosage of drug did the child receive?

13. Give erythromycin 75 mg P.O.

14. Give digoxin 0.125 mg P.O.

15. Give 100 mg V-cillin K P.O.

16. Read the V-cillin label. How many units comprise 1 mg?

17. Give 125 000 units of V-cillin K P.O.

18. Read the Lanoxin label. How many mcg are contained in 1.5 tabs?

19. What is the total amount of erythromycin in the bottle?

20. How many units of drug are there per mL of penicillin V potassium oral solution?

YOUR SCORE: _____ %

100%   YES — proceed to the next module
        NO — review this module or complete Appendix C

Note: if you had any errors on the posttest, analyze your areas of weakness.

Module 8: Dosage Calculations of Parenteral Medications

PRETEST

Instructions

1. Write the pretest without referring to any resource materials.

2. Correct the pretest using the answer guide.

3. If your score is 100 percent, you may wish to proceed to the next module.

4. If you do not achieve 100 percent, read the learning package in this module and complete the exercises, concentrating on your weak areas as diagnosed by your pretest score.

Calculate the following dosages:

Note: be careful to include the appropriate unit of measure with your answer, e.g., tablet, mg, mL. Round decimal numbers to the nearest hundredth.

1. The order is: heparin 8 000 units I.V. stat. The vial is labeled 10 000 units/mL. Determine the correct dose in mL.

2. The penicillin vial is labeled: 200 000 units/mL. The order is: 80 000 units I.M. Determine the correct dose in mL.

The order is: NPH insulin 22 units S.C. q.a.m. and regular insulin 12 units S.C. q.a.m. The vials are labeled: NPH 100 units/mL and regular 100 units/mL. Determine:

3. The correct dosage of NPH in mL

4. The correct dosage of regular in mL

5. The total dosage of insulin (the two insulins can be mixed in the same syringe)

6. The order is: perphenazine (Trilafon) 3.5 mg I.M. stat. The ampule is labeled 5 mg/mL. Determine the correct dosage in mL.

7. From hydrocortisone (Solu-Cortef) 100 mg/2 mL, determine the correct dosage for 75 mg I.M. daily.

8. The order is: meperidine (Demerol) 75 mg I.M. p.r.n. The ampule is labeled: meperidine 100 mg/ mL. Determine the correct dosage in mL.

For each of the following situations (questions 9 through 12), indicate whether the calculation is correct or incorrect.

9. The order is for heparin 5 000 units S.C. b.i.d. Available is heparin 10 000 units/mL. The correct dosage to administer subcutaneously is .5 mL.

10. The order is: dimenhydrinate (Gravol) 50 mg I.M. stat. The dosage available is an ampule labeled 50 mg/mL. The correct dosage to administer I.M. is 1 ampule.

11. Fluphenazine decanoate (Modecate) 12.5 mg I.M. is ordered. The vial is labeled:

    10 mL of Modecate
    25 mg/mL

The correct dosage to administer is 2 mL.

12. A colleague asks you to double-check the heparin dosage. The order is for 4 300 units I.V. by continuous infusion. The heparin is labeled 1 000 units/mL. Your colleague has drawn up 4 mL of heparin into a syringe. Is this correct?

13. You must administer 300 000 units of an antibiotic by I.M. injection. The label instructions state, "Add 5 mL of bacteriostatic water to yield 500 000 units per mL." Calculate the amount to give.

14. The order states: ampicillin 1 g I.V. q.6h. On hand is a vial of powdered medication. The label reads: 1 000 mg. If you add 1 mL of sterile water to the vial, calculate the dosage you will administer.

15. A multiple-dose vial containing a powdered antibiotic is labeled: Drug Q 10 g. The instructions state: add 7.2 mL of sterile water to yield 10 mL total volume. What is the concentration in g per mL?

16. Refer to question 15 and calculate a dose of 1 500 mg.

Refer to the drug labels on the facing page and answer questions 17 to 35.

For each of the following drug orders state the correct amount to administer. Be sure to state the dosage strength of the drug, for example, give 1 mL of the 10 mg/mL strength.

17. Prostaphlin 500 mg I.M. q.6h.

18. Morphine 10 mg I.M. q.3h.

19. Morphine 7.5 mg S.C. q.4h.

20. Prostaphlin 125 mg I.M. q.6h.

21. Morphine 12 mg to be added to an I.V. minibag and infused slowly.

22. You have drawn up 0.6 mL of morphine sulfate 10 mg/mL solution. How many mg is contained in this volume?

Complete the box below.

	Ancef	Prostaphlin	Polycillin-N
Volume of diluent	23.	24.	25.
Resulting concentration of solution	26.	27.	28.

29. Calculate 500 mg cefazolin sodium I.V.

30. Calculate 300 mg oxacillin sodium I.M.

YOUR SCORE: _____ %

100%   YES—proceed to the next module
        NO —complete this module

Note: if you had any errors on the pretest, analyze your areas of weakness.

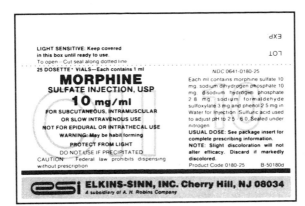

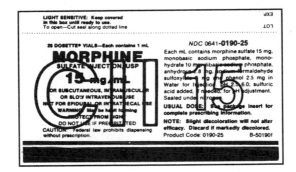

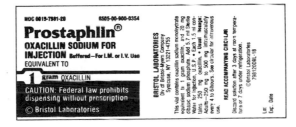

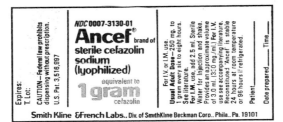

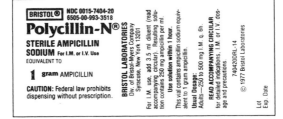

Learning Package

> **Objective**
> **To calculate dosages of**
> **parenteral medications**
> **accurately**

Before studying the calculation of liquid medications for parenteral administration, you should be familiar with the calibration of syringes. This module does not acquaint you with the procedure of injections. Examine the figures only to become familiar with the calibration of each type of syringe. Figure 8.1 illustrates a 2.5 mL syringe that is calibrated in 0.1 mL units. Figure 8.2 illustrates a 1-mL or 1-cc syringe that is calibrated in 0.01 mL units. (Recall from Module 5 that 1 mL = 1 cc.) If you aren't familiar with syringes, study these figures.

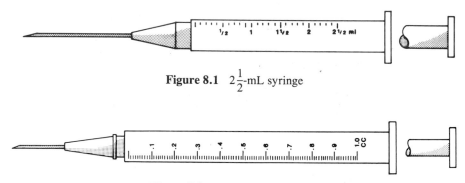

Figure 8.1 $2\frac{1}{2}$-mL syringe

Figure 8.2   1-mL or 1-cc syringe

The following example illustrates the calculation of a liquid medication for parenteral administration.

> Example:
>
> Ordered: 110 units of Drug M
> Available: Drug M 100 units/mL
>
> Known ratio: 100 units/1 mL
> Unknown ratio: 110 units/N mL
> 100:1 = 110:N
> 100 N = 110
>
> $N = \dfrac{100}{110} = 1.1$
>
> Answer is 1.1 mL

Figure 8-3 illustrates 1.1 mL in a 2.5-mL syringe.

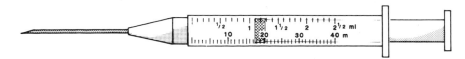

Figure 8.3 $2\frac{1}{2}$-mL syringe filled to 1.1 mL.

Exercise 8.1

Complete the following exercise without referring to the previous text. Correct using the answer guide. Be careful that the appropriate units are part of your answer. Include two places to the right of the decimal (hundredths) in your response.

1. The order is: heparin 7 500 units S.C. You have a 5-mL vial of heparin labeled: 10 000 units/mL. Determine the correct dosage to administer.

2. The label on a 2-mL ampule indicates 50 mg/mL. How many mg are contained in 1.5 mL?

3. The vial label states: add 3.5 mL of diluent: resulting solution contains 250 mg ampicillin per mL. Calculate 400 mg I.M.

4. Your patient has an order for meperidine (Demerol) 75 mg I.M. The 2-mL ampule is labeled: 50 mg/mL. How many mL should the patient receive?

5. The physician has ordered 0.1 mg of Medication A. The ampule is labeled: Medication A: 0.25 mg in 5 mL. Determine the correct dosage to administer.

For each of the following questions, shade in the accompanying syringe to indicate the correct dosage.

6. Ordered: heparin 5 000 units S.C.
   On hand: heparin 10 000 units/mL

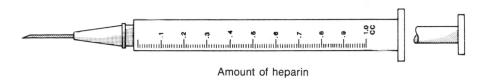

Amount of heparin

Figure 8.4   Amount of heparin.

7. Ordered: NPH insulin 37 units
   On hand: NPH insulin 100 units/mL

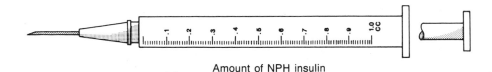

Amount of NPH insulin

Figure 8.5   Amount of NPH insulin.

8. Ordered: morphine 15 mg I.M. and perphenazine (Trilafon) 3.5 mg
   On hand: morphine 15 mg/mL and perphenazine 5 mg/mL
These two drugs can be mixed in the same syringe. Calculate the total amount.

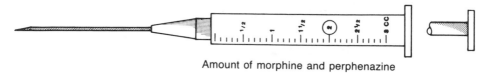

Amount of morphine and perphenazine

Figure 8.6 Amount of morphine and perphenazine.

9. Ordered: dimenhydrinate (Gravol) 30 mg I.M. p.r.n.
   On hand: 50 mg/mL

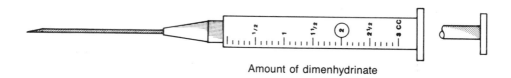

Amount of dimenhydrinate

Figure 8.7 Amount of dimenhydrinate.

10. An analgesic is ordered: 75 mg I.M. stat. On hand is a 2-mL ampule with a dosage concentration of 50 mg/mL. Calculate the dose to administer.

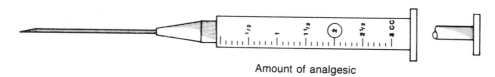

Amount of analgesic

Figure 8.8 Amount of analgesic.

Reconstituting Medications

To increase their stability, some medications are prepared in a dry powder form and must be diluted with a sterile solvent before administration. For example, many antibiotics must be reconstituted with sterile water. Refer to Table 8-A, which illustrates a dilution table on a multiple-dose vial. Note that adding 46 mL of sterile diluent yields a solution with 200 000 I.U. (International Units) of medication in each millilitre. Contrast this concentration with the solution that results when only 6 mL of diluent, usually sterile water, are added.

When a certain volume of liquid is added to a powdered drug in a vial, the resulting product will be of a greater volume. For example, adding 9.3 mL of fluid may result in a final volume in the vial of 10 mL. The powdered drug occupies some volume.

Table 8-A: Dilution

Potency Required I.U. per mL	Add Sterile Aqueous Diluent
200 000	46 mL
250 000	36 mL
750 000	9.3 mL
1 000 000	6 mL

Now study the labels below and on page 94 and be certain that you understand the following information before proceeding to Exercise 8.2.

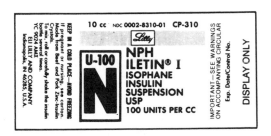

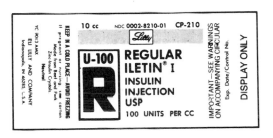

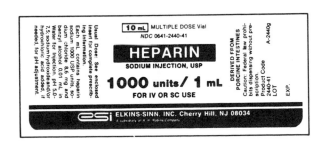

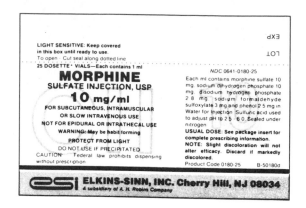

LIGHT SENSITIVE: Keep covered
in this box until ready to use.
To open · Cut seal along dotted line

ЕХР

ЛОТ

25 DOSETTE* VIALS—Each contains 1 ml

NDC 0641-0180-25

MORPHINE
SULFATE INJECTION, USP
10 mg/ml

FOR SUBCUTANEOUS, INTRAMUSCULAR
OR SLOW INTRAVENOUS USE
NOT FOR EPIDURAL OR INTRATHECAL USE
WARNING: May be habit forming
PROTECT FROM LIGHT
DO NOT USE IF PRECIPITATED
CAUTION   Federal law prohibits dispensing
without prescription

Each ml contains morphine sulfate 10
mg. sodium dihydrogen phosphate 10
mg. disodium hydrogen phosphate
2 8 mg sodium formaldehyde
sulfoxylate 3 mg and phenol 2 5 mg in
Water for Injection Sulfuric acid used
to adjust pH to 2 5 · 6 0. Sealed under
nitrogen

USUAL DOSE: See package insert for
complete prescribing information.
NOTE: Slight discoloration will not
alter efficacy. Discard if markedly
discolored.
Product Code 0180-25   B-50180d

ELKINS-SINN, INC. Cherry Hill, NJ 08034
A subsidiary of A. H. Robins Company

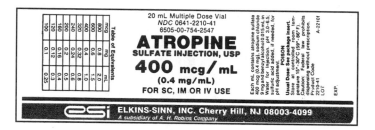

Table of Equivalents			
mcg	mg	ml	
100	0.1	0.25	
120	0.12	0.3	
160	0.16	0.4	
200	0.2	0.5	
240	0.24	0.6	
320	0.32	0.8	
400	0.4	1.0	
600	0.6	1.5	
800	0.8	2.0	

20 mL Multiple Dose Vial
NDC 0641-2210-41
6505-00-754-2547

ATROPINE
SULFATE INJECTION, USP
400 mcg/mL
(0.4 mg/mL)
FOR SC, IM OR IV USE

Each mL contains atropine sulfate
400 mcg (0.4 mg), sodium chloride
9 mg and benzyl alcohol 0.015mL in
Water for Injection, pH 3.0–6.5;
sulfuric acid added, if needed, for
pH adjustment.

POISON

Usual Dose: See package insert.
Store at controlled room tem-
perature 15°–30°C (59°–86°F)
Caution: Federal law prohibits
dispensing without prescription.
Product Code
2210-41
LOT
EXP.

A-2210f

ELKINS-SINN, INC. Cherry Hill, NJ 08003-4099
A subsidiary of A. H. Robins Company

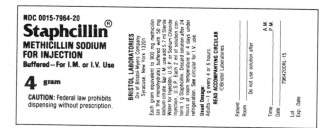

NDC 0015-7964-20

Staphcillin®
METHICILLIN SODIUM
FOR INJECTION
Buffered—For I.M. or I.V. Use

4 gram

CAUTION: Federal law prohibits
dispensing without prescription.

BRISTOL LABORATORIES
Div of Bristol-Myers Company
Syracuse, New York 13201

Each gram equivalent to 900 mg. methicillin
(as the monohydrate) buffered with 50 mg
sodium citrate. For I.M. use add 5.7 ml Sterile
Water for Injection, U.S.P. or Sodium Chloride
Injection, U.S.P. Each 2 ml of solution contains 1 g Staphcillin. Discard solution after 24
hours at room temperature or 4 days under
refrigeration. See circular for I.V. use.

Usual Dosage:
Adults—1 g every 4 or 6 hours.

READ ACCOMPANYING CIRCULAR
©Bristol Laboratories

Do not use solution after

A.M.
P.M.

Patient
Room

Time
Date

Lot   7964200RL-15
Exp. Date

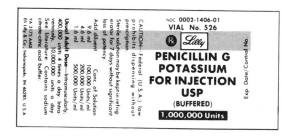

YA 3175 AMX
Eli Lilly & Co., Indianapolis, IN 46285, U.S.A.

Usual Adult Dose:—Intramuscularly,
400,000 units 4 times a day. Intravenously, 10,000,000 units a day.
See literature. Contains sodium
citrate-citric acid buffer.

Add diluent
9 ml
4.6 ml
1.6 ml

Conc. of Solution
100,000 Units/ml
200,000 Units/ml
500,000 Units/ml

Sterile solution may be kept in refrigerator for 7 days without significant
loss of potency.

CAUTION: Federal (U.S.A.) law
prohibits dispensing without
prescription.

NDC 0002-1406-01
VIAL No. 526

℞ Lilly

PENICILLIN G
POTASSIUM
FOR INJECTION
USP
(BUFFERED)

1,000,000 Units

Exp. Date/Control No.

For example, the pencillin G potassium vial contains 5 million units of pencillin G potassium. There are three options for reconstituting the powder and producing a solution of three different strengths. Adding 18 mL of diluent (the package instructions specify sterile water) will yield a solution with a strength (or concentration) of 250 000 units/mL. Continue reading the label. What is the concentration if you add 8 mL of diluent? 3 mL? Your answers should be 500 000 units/mL and 1 million units/mL. Now let's do several calculations using this vial label.

Example: the order is pencillin G potassium 750 000 units I.M. q.4h.

First reconstitute the solution by adding diluent. But how much should you add? Calculate using each option, then make your decision based on principles of drug administration by the I.M. route.

Option A

Add 18 mL of diluent for a solution concentration of 250 000 units/mL.
Solve: 250 000 units:1 mL = 750 000 units:N mL
$$250\ 000\ N = 750\ 000$$
$$N = 750\ 000/250\ 000$$
$$N = 3\ mL$$

Option B

Add 8 mL of diluent for a solution concentration of 500 000 units/mL
Solve: 500 000 units:1 mL = 750 000 units:N mL
$$N = 1.5\ mL.$$

Exercise 8.2

Refer to the vial label illustrated in Table 8-A to answer the following questions. Correct using the answer guide.

1. The order is for 750 000 units I.V. q.4h. How much diluent would you add to yield a solution with a concentration of 750 000 units/mL?

2. The medication has been mixed by another nurse and the vial is signed, dated, and marked to indicate that 9.3 mL of sterile diluent was added. How much would be required to administer a dose of 1 million units?

You add 46 mL of sterile diluent and mix the powdered drug. For each of the following orders indicate the correct volume to administer:

3. 750 000 units

4. 400 000 units

5. 250 000 units

You add 36 mL of sterile diluent and mix the powdered drug. For each of the following volumes, indicate the amount of drug (in units):

6. 1 mL

7. 0.8 mL

8. 1.4 mL

Refer to the vial labels on p. 94 and answer questions 9 to 15.

9. Give 1 000 000 units of penicillin G potassium I.V. (Describe the procedure for reconstitution.)

10. Give 400 000 units of penicillin G potassium I.M. (Describe the procedure for reconstitution.)

11. The penicillin G potassium vial has been reconstituted by adding 4.6 mL of diluent on the seventh day of the month at 1000 hours. Give 300 000 units I.M.

12. Refer to the previous question. On what day will this vial be outdated?

13. Give 1 g methicillin sodium I.M. (State the procedure for reconstitution.)

14. Give 750 mg staphcillin I.M. (State the procedure for reconstitution.)

15. Staphcillin is reconstituted on the twenty-first day at 0800 hours. When is it outdated, if stored in a refrigerator?

POSTTEST

Instructions

1. Write the posttest without referring to any reference materials.

2. Correct the posttest using the answer guide.

3. If your score is 100 percent, proceed to the next module.

4. If you do not achieve 100 percent, complete Appendix C or review the appropriate sections of the learning package in this module and rewrite the posttest.

5. Be careful to include units with all answers (e.g., mg, mL, tab). Round decimal numbers to the nearest hundredth.

1. A physician orders penicillin 400 000 units I.M. The label indicates penicillin 300 000 units/mL. Determine the correct dosage to give.

2. Oxytetracycline hydrochloride (Terramycin) 0.3 g is ordered I.M.; the vial is labeled 100 mg/mL. How many mL should you give?

Refer to the labels on pages 93–94 and answer questions 3 to 25.

3. The physician orders 25 units of NPH insulin. Determine the correct dosage.

The order is: 35 units NPH insulin and 15 units of regular insulin Calculate the following:

4. The volume of NPH insulin required

5. The volume of regular insulin required

6. The total volume that should be drawn up in one syringe (these two insulins are mixed and administered in the same syringe).

7. Your patient is learning to administer her insulin. The order is for 22 units of NPH and 8 units of regular insulin. She asks you to check her dosage. The syringe markings indicate that she has drawn up 0.3 mL. Is this correct?

8. The physician has ordered penicillin G potassium 600 000 units I.M. How many mL should the patient receive? State the procedure for reconstitution.

The order is: morphine 8 mg I.M. and atropine sulfate 0.4 mg I.M. 1 hour preoperatively. Calculate:

9. The dosage of morphine

10. The dosage of atropine

11. The total volume in the syringe after the two drugs are drawn up. (These drugs can be mixed together for a short time.)

12. Calculate heparin 2 500 units.

The label on the penicillin G potassium indicates that 9.6 mL of diluent was added at 1300 hours on the seventeenth day of the month. Answer questions 13 to 15.

13. State the concentration of the solution.

14. Calculate 250 000 units I.M. stat.

15. State the hour and day of the month the drug is outdated.

16. Add morphine 10 mg to a 100-mL bag of I.V. solution. State the volume of morphine required and the concentration of the I.V. solution.

Complete the box below.

	Penicillin G potassium	Methicillin sodium
Shelf life after reconstitution	17.	18.
Route of administration	19.	20.
Total amount of drug in vial	21.	22.

23. Calculate this insulin order: regular insulin 8 units and NPH insulin 28 units S.C.

24. Give atropine 0.3 mg S.C.

25. Calculate staphcillin 1 g I.M.

Refer to the following order for questions 26 to 28. State the procedure for reconstitution.

The order is: 500 000 units I.V. q.6h. You have on hand a 10-mL vial that is labeled 10 000 000 units. Calculate:

26. The concentration of drug per mL

27. The volume required to administer the dose ordered

28. The number of dosages this vial contains (for the amount ordered for this patient)

Refer to the syringes below and answer questions 29 and 30.

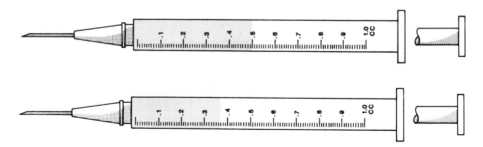

29. The vial label states heparin 1 000 units/mL. How many units of heparin are contained in syringe A?

30. The vial label states heparin 10 000 units/mL. How many units are contained in syringe B?

YOUR SCORE: _____ %

100%   YES — proceed to the next module
         NO — review this module or complete Appendix C

Note: if you had any errors on the posttest, analyze your areas of weakness.

Module 9: Intravenous Administration

PRETEST

Instructions

1. Write the pretest without referring to any resource materials.

2. Correct the pretest using the answer guide.

3. Be careful to:
   a. include the appropriate units of measure with the answer when necessary
   b. round decimal numbers to nearest whole number
   c. write decimal numbers correctly, using a zero to the left of the decimal point when necessary

You should deduct marks if your answers aren't expressed correctly, as indicated above.

4. If your score is 100 percent, you are ready for the "real world" of calculating most medications for administration to patients in the clinical setting — assuming, of course, that you have mastered the preceding modules.

5 If you don't achieve 100 percent accuracy, read the learning package in this module and complete the exercises, concentrating on your weak areas as diagnosed by your pretest score.

For each of the following clinical situations, calculate as directed:

Order 1: the patient is to receive 1 L of I.V. fluid in 8 hours.

1. For order 1, calculate the number of mL per minute that the patient should receive.

2. For order 1, calculate the rate of flow in drops per minute (the drop factor is 10).

3. A 500-mL I.V. is infusing at the rate of 25 mL per hour. How many hours will it take for this I.V. to be infused?

Order 2: 1 L q.12h.

4. For order 2, calculate the volume to be infused in 1 hour.

5. For order 2, calculate the rate of flow using a minidrip set (the drop factor is 60).

6. Ampicillin has been added to 50 mL of normal saline. The drug should be infused in 20 minutes. Calculate the rate of flow using a regular set with a drop factor of 1 mL = 10 drops.

Order 3: 2 L/day.

7. For order 3, calculate the hourly rate of infusion.

8. For order 3, calculate the drip rate (the drop factor is 60).

9. The order is for 1 500 mL of saline over 24 hours. Calculate the infusion rate per minute if the administration set delivers 10 drops/mL.

10. A litre of I.V. fluid has been running at 125 mL/hour for 3.5 hours. How much remains in the I.V. container?

11. The I.V. is ordered to run at 50 mL/hour. The administration set delivers 60 drops/mL. Calculate the infusion rate in drops per minute.

12. The I.V. container is labeled: "infuse at 100 mL/hour." The administration set delivers 10 drops/mL. The I.V. is running at a rate of 20 drops per minute. Is this correct?

13. An I.V. container of 500 mL has infused for 1 hour at a rate of 100 mL/hour. A new rate of infusion is ordered at 50 mL/hour. Calculate the number of hours during which the remaining fluid will infuse.

14. The order is for 500 mL of blood over 3 hours. Calculate the rate of flow using a set with a drop factor of 15.

15. The I.V. is infusing at 125 drops per minute with a minidrip (the drop factor is 60). How long will it take to infuse 250 mL?

16. A medication is ordered for I.V. administration. The order is for 200 mg and the drug is available as 200 mg in 50 mL solution. The infusion set delivers 60 drops/mL. The drug is to infuse in 30 minutes. Calculate the rate of flow in drops per minute.

17. Nafcillin sodium (Unipen) 0.5 g I.V. q.6h is ordered. The admixture from the pharmacy contains nafcillin sodium 500 mg in a 100-mL bag. The infusion set delivers 10 drops/mL. Calculate the drip rate if the drug is to infuse in 30 minutes.

18. An I.V. piggyback with 500 mg of drug in 50 mL of solution is infusing at a rate of 100 mL/hour. How much drug is infused in 15 minutes?

19. The order is for 250 mg ampicillin I.V. stat and the pharmacy is closed. Available is a 250-mg vial for reconstitution. The package insert provides these instructions: add 2 mL of diluent to 250-mg vial to reconstitute; inject slowly over at least 10 to 15 minutes. Add ampicillin to 25 mL of I.V. solution and calculate the rate of flow if the set delivers 20 drops/mL.

20. Cephalothin sodium concentration is 1 g in 100 mL of solution. The accompanying literature recommends infusing the drug over 30 minutes. Calculate the rate of flow for an infusion set of 15 drops/mL.

YOUR SCORE: _____ %

100%   YES — proceed to the next module
NO — complete this module

Note: if you had any errors on the pretest, analyze your areas of weakness.

Learning Package

```
               Objective
   To calculate the rate of flow
   of  intravenous  infusions
   using various drop factors
   accurately
```

Calculating Rate of Flow of Intravenous Infusions

All intravenous fluids and medications must be administered precisely. The desired rate of flow must be calculated accurately and observed frequently during I.V. therapy.

The volume and type of I.V. fluid is ordered by the physician. The safe rate of administration of I.V. fluids and medications is determined by many factors, including:

1. Age; infants and the elderly tolerate less fluid

2. Cardiovascular status

3. Site of infusion

4. Nature of the infusion; for example, irritating fluids or medications must be infused slowly to allow for adequate hemodilution

5. B.S.A., body surface area; the maximum rate of flow should not exceed 3 mL per square metre

I.V. fluids are administered either by infusion pumps or by gravity drip. When a pump is used the rate of flow is expressed in mL per hour. For gravity drip, the rate must be calculated in drops per minute. This requires an additional step in the calculation. This module focuses on clinical situations involving gravity drip. Figure 9.1 illustrates I.V. administration sets.

To calculate the rate of flow for a gravity drip, you must know the following:

1. The ordered rate of flow that must be converted to drops per minute to regulate the I.V. administration set

2. The calibration of the administration set in drops per mL; different sets are unique in this factor

Note: formula for dosage calculation is given in Appendix F.

```
Example:
administer 1 L of 5% dextrose q.8h.
Step 1. Convert order to mL/minute
Volume of fluid in mL = 1 L = 1 000 mL
Time in minutes = 8 × 60 = 480 minutes

 1 000 mL
──────────── = 2.1 mL/minute
480 minutes
```

> Step 2. Convert mL to drops/minute
> The intravenous tubing set delivers 10 drops/mL.
> Known ratio: 10 drops:1 mL
> Unknown ratio: N drops:2.1 mL
> 10 drops:1 mL = N drops:2.1 mL
> N = 21
> Answer: set roller clamp to allow 21 drops per minute.

Validate your answer:

$$\frac{1\,L}{8\,hours} = \frac{1\,000\,mL}{480\,minutes} = \frac{2.1\,mL}{minute} = \frac{21\,drops}{minute}$$

Not all I.V. sets deliver the same size of drops. It is essential that you determine the type of drip chamber being used. A minidrip delivers approximately 60 drops/mL. The previous calculation would differ considerably if a minidrip infusion set were used.

> Example: using a minidrip for the previous order
>
> Step 1. Convert order to mL/minute
> As in previous example, 1 L/8 hours = 2.1 mL/minute.
>
> Step 2. Convert to drops per minute
> Known ratio: 60 drops:1 mL
> Unknown ratio: N drops:2.1 mL
> 60 drops: 1 mL = N drops:2.1 mL
> N = 126
> Answer: set roller clamp to allow 126 drops per minute

Exercise 9.1

Complete the following exercise without referring to the previous text. Correct using the answer guide.

1. Order: 1 L of normal saline q.12h. Calculate the rate of flow using a minidrip with a drop factor of 60 drops/mL.

2. Order: 1 000 mL of two-thirds/one-third to run at 50 drops per minute. How many hours should this litre infuse using a minidrip (the drop factor is 60)?

Order: 3 000 mL of 5% dextrose over 24 hours.

3. For this order, calculate the rate of flow using a regular set (the drop factor is 10).

4. For this order, calculate the rate of flow using a minidrip set (the drop factor is 60).

5. The blood transfusion is infusing at 25 drops per minute, and the set is calibrated at 15 drops/mL. What is the hourly infusion rate, in mL?

Order: administer 3 000 mL/sq m × 24 hours. The patient's body surface area in square metres is 1.2. (The concept of body surface area is discussed in Module 10, but the arithmetic principles should be clear to you.)

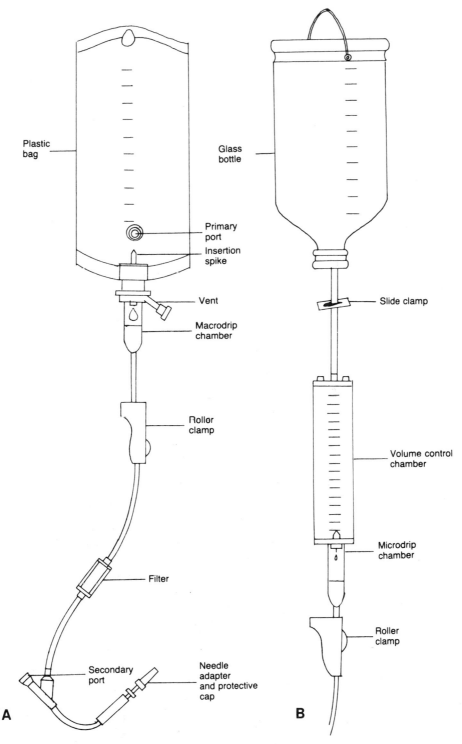

Figure 9.1   I.V. administration sets. **A**, Regular drip (macrodrip). **B**, Minidrip (microdrip). (From Clayton, B.D., and others: Squire's basic pharmacology for nurses, ed. 8, St. Louis, 1985, The C.V. Mosby Co.)

6. For this order, calculate the total amount of fluid to infuse in 24 hours.

7. For this order, calculate the hourly infusion rate.

8. For this order, calculate the rate in drops per minute using a regular drip infusion set (the drop factor is 10).

9. The ordered dose of methotrexate is dissolved in 1 L to be infused over 1 hour. Calculate the rate of flow in drops per minute using a regular drip set (the drop factor is 10).

10. The order is to infuse normal saline with an antineoplastic drug, over 6 hours. Using a regular drip, with a drop factor of 10, calculate the rate of flow in drops per minute.

Calculating Fluid Needs

Fluids may be ordered as L/day or mL/hour or according to body weight or body surface area. For children, the recommended fluid replacement is 1 500 mL/sq m/day. The following calculation illustrates these concepts.

Calculate the hourly fluid replacement rate for a child with body surface area of 0.6 sq m.

Solution

1 500 mL per sq m for this child = 1 500 × 0.6 = 900 mL. This child should receive 900 mL of fluid per day. Here's how to express the solution as an hourly rate:

$$\frac{900}{24} = 37.5 \text{ or } 38 \text{ mL/hour}$$

Another guide used for both children and adults is the following:

100 mL/kg for the first 10 kg
50 mL/kg for the next 10 kg
20 mL/kg for the next 20 or more kg

> Example: calculate the 24-hour fluid needs for an individual weighing 60 kg
>
> For the first 10 kg: 100 mL/kg = 1 000 mL
> For the next 10 kg: 50 mL/kg = 500 mL
> For the remaining 40 kg: 20 mL/kg = 20 × 40 = 800 mL
> Total: 1 000 + 500 + 800 = 2 300 mL/24 hours

Calculating Kilojoules

Sometimes you need to keep track of the kilojoules received in I.V. fluids. In a 5% dextrose solution, for example, every 100 mL of solution contains 5 g of dextrose. Each g of dextrose supplies 11.3 kilojoules (or 3.4 K calories).

Exercise 9.2

Complete the exercise by using the guidelines above. Validate your responses, then correct using the answer guide.

Calculate the daily fluid needs for each of the following individuals:

1. A man weighing 209 pounds
2. A girl weighing 42 pounds
3. A child weighing 12 pounds, 4 oz
4. A woman weighing 50 kg
5. A teenager weighing 57 kg

Calculate the total kilojoules supplied in a 24-hour period for each of the following individuals, assuming that 5% dextrose solution is used. Round your answer to the nearest whole number.

6. A man weighing 209 pounds
7. A girl weighing 42 pounds
8. A child weighing 12 pounds, 4 oz
9. A woman weighing 50 kg
10. A teenager weighing 57 kg

Intravenous Medications

Today many medications are administered by the I.V. route, which ensures complete absorption of the drug and rapid action. Medications may be premixed in the I.V. solution, added to the solution by the nurse, or administered by ''piggyback''; where the drug is added to a small volume of fluid (50 to 200 mL) in a minibag or buretrol and infused over a short time. The principles of calculation are the same: determine the dosage of medication, add it to the I.V. solution, and calculate the rate of flow. The following exercise provides practice.

Exercise 9.3

Complete the following exercise and correct using the answer guide.

For problems 1 to 4 use a minidrip administration set; the drop factor is 60 drops/mL.

1. Kanamycin sulfate (Kantrex) 500 mg in 200 mL of normal saline infused over 2.5 hours
   a. Calculate the flow rate in drops per minute.
   b. How much of the drug (in mg) is delivered per minute?

2. Give cefazolin sodium 250 mg I.V. q.8h. Dilute in 50 mL of normal saline and infuse in 30 minutes.
   a. Calculate the flow rate in drops per minute.
   b. How much drug (in mg) is delivered per minute?

3. Cephalothin sodium 4 g to be infused over 1 hour. Reconstitute the powdered drug with 20 mL of sterile water and add to a 100-mL minibag of D-5-W. Calculate the rate of flow in drops per minute.

4. Calculate the rate of flow in drops per minute for ampicillin 500 mg in 50 mL infused in 20 minutes.

5. Penicillin 500 000 units is added to 100 mL; the rate of administration is ordered at 125 mL per hour. Using an infusion set with a drop factor of 20 drops/mL, calculate:
  a. The rate of flow in drops per minute
  b. The time to infuse the drug

6. Heparin 4 000 units q.4h. by continuous I.V. using a 100-mL minibag, microdrip (60 drops/mL), and heparin 10 000 units/mL, calculate:
  a. The amount of heparin solution to add to the minibag
  b. The rate of flow in drops per minute

Refer to the labels on the opposite page and answer questions 7 to 15.

7. Ordered: gentamycin sulfate 70 mg I.V. q.8h.; the I.V. rate of flow is 50 mL/hour. A 50-mL minibag and microdrip infusion set (60 drops/mL) are available. Calculate:
  a. The amount of drug to add to the minibag
  b. The rate of flow in drops per minute

8. Order: 250 mg cefazolin sodium I.V. q.8h; the instructions in the package insert state to dilute the drug in 50 mL of normal saline. The current I.V. is infusing at 125 mL/hour. Calculate:
  a. The current rate of flow in drops per minute using a microdrip (60 drops/mL)
  b. The amount of cefazolin sodium required
  c. If the drug is started at 1300 hours, at what time will it be infused?

9. Cephalothin sodium 500 mg I.V. q.4h. infused over 1 hour; the current I.V. is infusing at 75 mL/hour
  a. Describe reconstitution.
  b. Calculate the dosage.
  c. State the volume that the drug is added to and the rate of flow in drops per minute using an infusion set with a drop factor of 15.

10. Order: oxacillin sodium 0.5 g q.6h.
  a. How many doses can be obtained from the vial illustrated?
  b. Add the drug to a 100-mL minibag and infuse over 1 hour; calculate the rate of flow in drops per minute; the drop factor is 20.

11. The order is for methicillin sodium 1 g q.6h. in 50 mL NS; infuse at 10 mL/minute
  a. Describe reconstitution.
  b. Calculate the dosage.
  c. Calculate the rate of flow in drops per minute; use an infusion set with a drop factor of 10.

12. Which drugs illustrated in these labels must be discarded 24 hours after reconstitution if left at room temperature?

Medications can be administered directly into a vein (called bolus injections). Usually they must be diluted, then given over 2 to 5 minutes. For each of the following situations, indicate the amount of sterile water that must be added to obtain the desired concentration.

Drug	Available Concentration	Desired Concentration	Amount of Sterile Water to Add
A	10 mg/mL	2 mg/mL	13.
B	0.5 mg/mL	100 mcg/mL	14.
C	10 mg/5 mL	1 mg/mL	15.

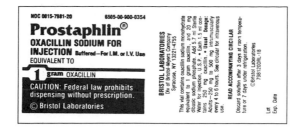

NDC 0015-7981-20   6505-00-900-0354

Prostaphlin®
OXACILLIN SODIUM FOR
INJECTION Buffered—For I.M. or I.V. Use
EQUIVALENT TO

1 gram OXACILLIN

CAUTION: Federal law prohibits
dispensing without prescription.
© Bristol Laboratories

BRISTOL LABORATORIES
Div of Bristol-Myers Company
Syracuse, NY 13221-4755

This vial contains oxacillin sodium monohydrate
equivalent to 1 gram oxacillin, and 20 mg
dibasic sodium phosphate. Add 5.7 ml Sterile
Water for Injection, U.S.P. • Each 1.5 ml contains 250 mg oxacillin. • **Usual Dosage:**
Adults—250 mg to 500 mg intramuscularly
every 4 to 6 hours. See circular for intravenous
use.

READ ACCOMPANYING CIRCULAR

Discard solution after 3 days at room temperature or 7 days under refrigeration.

©Bristol Laboratories
7981200RL-18

Lot
Exp. Date

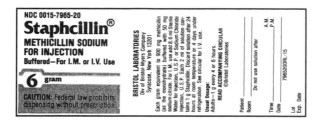

NDC 0015-7965-20

Staphcillin®
METHICILLIN SODIUM
FOR INJECTION
Buffered—For I.M. or I.V. Use

6 gram

CAUTION: Federal law prohibits
dispensing without prescription.

BRISTOL LABORATORIES
Div of Bristol-Myers Company
Syracuse, New York 13201

Each gram equivalent to 900 mg methicillin
(as the monohydrate) buffered with 50 mg
sodium citrate. For I.M. use add 8.6 ml Sterile
Water for Injection, U.S.P. Each 2 ml of solution contains 1 g Staphcillin. Discard solution after 24
hours at room temperature or 4 days under
refrigeration. See circular for I.V. use.

Usual Dosage:
Adults—1 g every 4 or 6 hours.

READ ACCOMPANYING CIRCULAR

©Bristol Laboratories

Patient
Room   Do not use solution after
                                              A.M.
                                              P.M.
Time
Date   7965200RL-15
Lot
Exp. Date

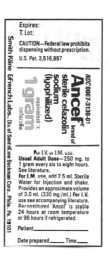

NDC 2-N57-1
AMPOULE No. 698

℞ *Lilly*

KEFLIN®
STERILE SODIUM
CEPHALOTHIN, U.S.P.

Equivalent to **1 Gm.** Cephalothin
To prepare I.M. solution add **4 ml.** of
Sterile Water for Injection SHAKE WELL
Provides two 0.5 Gm doses of 2.2 ml each
For I.V. solution see literature

XU 0143 AMX
Eli Lilly & Co. Indianapolis, Ind. 46206, U.S.A
Exp. Date

Usual Adult Dose—2 to 12 Gm. daily. See literature.
After Reconstitution When refrigerated, the solution has a satisfactory potency for 48 hours. Kept
at room temperature, in ambocular solutions
should be used in injection solutions should be sterile
intermittent I.V. infusion should be sterile
within 6 hours and completed within 24 hours. For
prolonged infusions replace with a fresh prepared solution at least every 24 hours.

Patient
Date Prepared
Time

Expires:
T. Lot:

CAUTION—Federal law prohibits
dispensing without prescription.

U.S. Pat. 3,516,997

NDC 0007-3130-01
Ancef®
brand of
sterile cefazolin
sodium
(lyophilized)

1 gram
equivalent to

Smith Kline &French Labs., Div. of SmithKline Beckman Corp., Phila., Pa. 19101

For I.V. or I.M. use.
Usual Adult Dose—250 mg. to
1 gram every six to eight hours.
See literature.
For I.M. use, add 2.5 ml. Sterile
Water for Injection and shake.
Provides an approximate volume
of 3.0 ml. (330 mg./ml.) **For I.V.**
use see accompanying literature.
Reconstituted 'Ancef' is stable
24 hours at room temperature
or 96 hours if refrigerated.

Patient

Date prepared_____ Time____

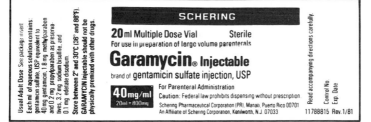

Usual Adult Dose See package insert

Each ml of aqueous solution contains:
gentamicin sulfate, USP equivalent to
40 mg gentamicin, 1.8 mg methylparaben
and 0.2 mg propylparaben as a preserva-
tives, 3.2 mg sodium bisulfite, and
0.1 mg edetate disodium

Store between 2° and 30°C (36° and 86°F).
GARAMYCIN Injectable should not be
physically premixed with other drugs.

SCHERING

20 ml Multiple Dose Vial   Sterile
For use in preparation of large volume parenterals

Garamycin® Injectable
brand of gentamicin sulfate injection, USP

40 mg/ml
20ml = 800mg

For Parenteral Administration
Caution: Federal law prohibits dispensing without prescription.
Schering Pharmaceutical Corporation (PR). Manati, Puerto Rico 00701
An Affiliate of Schering Corporation, Kenilworth, N.J 07033

Read accompanying directions carefully.

Control No
Exp. Date

11788815 Rev.1/81

POSTTEST

Instructions

1. Write the posttest without referring to any reference materials.

2. Correct the posttest using the answer guide.

3. Be careful to:
   a. Include the appropriate units of measure with the answer when necessary
   b. Round decimal numbers to the nearest whole number
   c. Write decimal numbers correctly, using a zero to the left of the decimal point when necessary

   You should deduct marks if your answers are not expressed correctly, as indicated above.

4. If your score is 100 percent, congratulations! You are ready for the "real world" of calculating most medications for administration to patients in the clinical setting — assuming, of course, that you have mastered the preceding modules. Module 10 explains more complex but less common clinical calculations. You will want to proceed to this module before practicing in the following settings: pediatrics, coronary or extra care units, emergency, and neonatal units.

5. If you don't achieve 100 percent, review the learning package in this module and rewrite the posttest.

For each of the following clinical situations, calculate as directed:

Order 1: 1 000 mL q.8h.

1. For order 1, calculate the rate of flow using a minidrip with a drop factor of 60.

2. For order 1, calculate the rate of flow using a set with a drop factor of 10.

Order 2: aminophylline 50 mg per hour, to be given by continuous infusion. The intravenous manual instructions are as follows: "dilute to a concentration of 1 mg/mL of dextrose or normal saline."

3. For order 2, calculate the volume of fluid required for a 2-hour infusion.

4. For order 2, calculate the rate of flow using a minidrip set (the drop factor is 60).

5. For order 2, a 50-mL minibag is marked in this way: "contains 50 mg of aminophylline." It is infusing at 50 drops per minute (the drop factor is 60). How much of the drug is infused in 30 minutes?

6. For order 2, calculate the length of time to infuse this drug if 500 mg is added to 500 mL and a minidrip set is used (the drop factor is 60).

Order 3: ampicillin 250 mg q.6h. The patient has an I.V. infusing with a minidrip set (the drop factor is 60). The intravenous manual instructions are: "dilute to 5 mg/mL and infuse over 30 minutes."

7. For order 3, calculate the volume of fluid required to dilute the drug.

8. For order 3, calculate the rate of flow.

Order 4: 1 000 mL q.8h. × 24 hours. After 3 hours, with a regular set (the drop factor is 10), only 300 mL are absorbed.

9. For order 4, calculate the volume that should have infused in the 3-hour period.

10. For order 4, calculate the new rate of flow for the remaining 700 mL to be absorbed within the ordered time period.

11. Calculate the rate of flow (the drop factor is 10) for this order: "500 mL over 3 hours."

12. Using an administration set with a drop factor of 15 and an infusion rate of 15 drops per minute, how much time would be required to infuse 60 mL?

13. A 100-mL minibag infusing at 50 drops per minute (the drop factor is 60) is initiated at 1000 hours. At what time should it be completely infused?

14. An I.V. is infusing at 125 mL per hour. How many mL will be absorbed in a 12-hour shift?

15. An I.V. infuses at 20 drops per minute (the drop factor is 10) for 4 hours. How much has infused?

16. Order: cefoperazone sodium 1 g q.12h. I.V. A 2-g vial is available; the instructions state: add 19 mL of diluent to achieve a volume of 20 mL and concentration of 100 mg/mL; may be added to I.V. infusion solutions and administered by intermittent or continuous infusion. I.V. of D-5-W is infusing at 1 L q.8h. Calculate the following:

    a. The amount of cefoperazone sodium required for one dose; describe reconstitution

    b. The rate of flow of the I.V. if the infusion set drop factor is 20 drops/mL

    c. The volume of I.V. fluid required to maintain the above flow rate and to infuse the drug over 30 minutes

17. Order: cephalothin sodium loading dose of 2 g I.V. before surgery; a vial stating that it contains 2 g of cephalothin with 63 mg of sodium per gram is available. The instructions are to dilute the drug with 20 mL of sterile water for injection, then add it to the intravenous infusion. The I.V. of normal saline is infusing at 100 mL/hour. Calculate the following:

    a. The required amount of cephalothin sodium for the loading dose; describe reconstitution

    b. The rate of flow of the I.V. if the infusion set delivers 10 drops/mL

    c. The amount of sodium the patient will receive with the loading dose

    d. Maintain the original rate of flow of the I.V. infusion and state the volume of I.V. fluid to dilute the cephalothin sodium dose and infuse it over 1 hour

18. Heparin 5 000 units q.8h. by continuous intravenous infusion. Available: a vial labeled heparin 10 000 units/mL. An I.V. of normal saline is infusing at 125 mL/hour. Calculate the following:

    a. The rate of flow in drops per minute if the infusion set drop factor is 60 drops/mL

    b. The volume of heparin required per dose

    c. The volume of I.V. solution used to provide continuous infusion for 8 hours

    d. The amount of drug infused per minute

19. Dosage ordered: 250 mg I.V. over 30 minutes q.4h. Available: a vial labeled 250 mg/100 mL. The drop factor is 10 drops/mL. Calculate:

    a. The volume of drug required for a single dose

    b. The rate of flow in drops per minute

20. Ordered: ampicillin 500 mg I.V. q.4h. Available: admixture solution of ampicillin 500 mg in a 50-mL bag. The infusion drop factor is 60 drops/mL. The drug should infuse in 30 minutes; the I.V. is infusing at 125 mL/hour. Calculate:

    a. The rate of flow in drops per minute for the main I.V. solution
    b. The rate of flow to infuse the drug
    c. The amount of ampicillin the patient will receive in 24 hours
    d. The volume of fluid infused in 24 hours; note the two rates of infusion, one for the drug and another to infuse the I.V. solution

YOUR SCORE: _____ %

100%   YES — proceed to the next module if you wish to do
               more complex calculations
      NO — review this module

Note: if you had any errors on the posttest, analyze your areas of weakness.

Module 10: Calculations for Children and Critical Care

PRETEST

Instructions

1. Write the pretest without referring to any resource materials.

2. Express decimal numbers rounded to the nearest tenth except rate of flow in drops per minute: express in whole numbers.

3. Correct the pretest using the answer guide.

4. If your score is 100 percent, congratulations! You have finished the workbook, assuming that you proceeded through the modules in sequence.

5. If you don't achieve 100 percent accuracy, read the learning package in this module and complete the exercises, concentrating on your weak areas as diagnosed by your pretest score.

Note: this module is designed to test advanced skills in dosage calculation. Don't proceed if you are faint-hearted. If you do proceed, don't be discouraged if you diagnose weaknesses in your ability to calculate intravenous administration of medications. This is a very challenging area, as any health professional in an acute care setting will agree.

Refer to this formula to calculate doses for children:

$$\text{Child's dose} = \frac{\text{B.S.A.}}{1.73\,\text{sq m}} \times \text{Adult dose}$$

1. Calculate the dose to be administered:
     Ordered: 10 mcg/kg epinephrine S.C. stat
     Available: epinephrine 1:1 000 = 1 mg/mL
     Child weighs 10 kg

2. An antibiotic is ordered: 2 g per square metre (body surface area). A child's B.S.A. is 0.45 sq m. Calculate the dose to administer.

3. Use the formula to calculate the dose for a child with a B.S.A. of 0.2 sq m if the usual adult dose is 60 mg.

4. Calculate the dose for a child with a B.S.A. of 1 sq m if the usual adult dose is 250 mg.

5. Calculate the dose for a child with a B.S.A. of 0.86 sq m if the usual adult dose is 50 mg.

6. State the concentration of medication in mcg per mL if 400 mg of the drug are added to 500 mL of I.V. solution.

7. Using an infusion set with a drop factor of 60 drops/mL, calculate the rate of flow in drops per minute to deliver 200 mcg/minute with the I.V. solution described in question 6.

8. State the concentration in mg/mL if 1 g of medication is added to 250 mL of I.V. solution.

9. Calculate the rate of infusion in drops per minute for this order: dopamine (Intropin) 3 mcg/kg/minute for a patient weighing 70 kg. Use a minibag containing 200 mg dopamine in 250 mL and a minidrip infusion set with a drop factor of 60 drops/mL.

Order 1: give 2 mcg/kg/minute I.V.

10. For order 1, calculate the dosage required for a patient weighing 65 kg.

11. For order 1, calculate the drug concentration in mcg/mL if 200 mg of drug is added to 250 mL of I.V. fluid.

12. For order 1, calculate the rate of flow in drops per minute using a minidrip infusion set with a drop factor of 60/mL and the drug concentration specified in question 11.

13. An I.V. minibag admixture is prepared with 1 mg of isoproterenol (Isuprel) in 250 mL of solution. Calculate the number of mcg/mL.

14. The drug is ordered as 5 mg per sq m. What is the dose for an individual with a B.S.A. of 1.3 sq m?

15. If 50 mg of a drug is added to 250 mL of I.V. solution, how much of the drug does the patient receive per minute at a rate of 60 drops per minute (when the drop factor is 60)?

Refer to the labels below and answer questions 16 to 20.

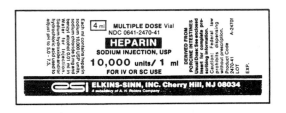

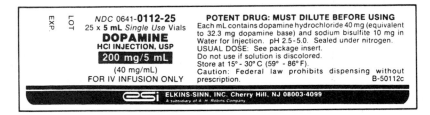

16. One litre of D-5-W with 30 000 units of heparin is to infuse at 40 mL/hour. Calculate:
   a. The volume of heparin to add to the I.V. solution
   b. The rate of flow using a minidrip (60 drops/mL)
   c. The dosage of the drug the patient receives per hour

17. A new order for question 16 states: increase the I.V. rate of flow to 50 mL/hour. Calculate the dosage of heparin that the patient receives per hour.

18. A new order for question 16 states: change the heparin dosage to 1 000 units per hour. Calculate the new rate of flow in mL/hour and drops/minute.

19. A patient weighing 59 kg has been admitted to the CCU. Order: infuse dopamine 5 mcg/kg/ minute. Prepare a 250-mL bag of I.V. solution containing dopamine with a concentration of 1 mg/mL. Calculate:

    a. The volume of dopamine to add to the I.V. bag
    b. The dose required per minute
    c. The rate of flow of the I.V. to deliver this dose if a minidrip set is used (60 drops/mL)

20. For the situation in question 19, calculate a new rate of flow to deliver 4 mcg/kg/minute.

YOUR SCORE: _____ %

100%   YES—Bravo! You have excellent skill in calculating dosages
           NO —complete this module

Note: if you had any errors on the pretest, analyze your areas of weakness.

Learning Package

> **Objective**
> **To calculate fractional dosages based on body weight or body surface area (B.S.A.) accurately**

In every clinical situation involving medication administration, accurate dosage calculation is an important responsibility. However, in some situations it is essential to patient safety. Neonatal, pediatric, elderly, and acutely-ill patients require very precise dosage administration.

This module doesn't present any new mathematical principles but provides practice in more complex dosage calculations, using body weight, body surface area, and dosages delivered by the I.V. route.

Calculating Dosages for Children

There are several "rules" that have been used in the past to calculate pediatric drug dosages. These rules are described in Appendix D. They were based on the child's age and the "average" adult dose. Today many references indicate the recommended dosages for children. If these aren't known, it is recognized practice to calculate pediatric dosages based on body weight or body surface area, because of the now accepted truth that children are not just "small adults." Therefore this module, in keeping with modern practice, will not discuss the old rules but will provide practice in calculating dosages based on body weight and body surface area.

Calculations Based on Body Weight

Dosages may be based on body weight and expressed as dose per kg, for example, mg/kg. The "desired dose" must first be calculated.

Example:

The order states: "give 1 mg/kg q.6h."
The available dosage strength is: 100 mg/mL.

Calculate the dosage for each of the following:
   a. A child weighing 20 kg
   b. An adult weighing 72 kg
   c. An adult weighing 61 kg

The dose desired for each patient is:
   a. 1 mg × 20 kg = 20 mg
   b. 1 mg × 72 kg = 72 mg
   c. 1 mg × 61 kg = 61 mg

Now use a proportion equation to determine each patient's dose.

Solution for Situation a

Known ratio: 100 mg:1 mL
Unknown ratio: 20 mg:N mL
100:1 = 20:N
100 N = 20
100 N (÷ 100) = 20 (÷ 100)
N = 0.2
Answer: give 0.2 mL

Solution for Situation b

100 mg:1 mL = 72 mg:N mL
100 N = 72
100 N (÷ 100) = 72 (÷ 100)
N = 0.72
Answer: give 0.72 mL

Solution for Situation c

100 mg:1 mL = 61 mg:N mL
100 N = 61
100 N (÷ 100) = 61 (÷ 100)
N = 0.61
Answer: give 0.61 mL

Example:

The order is: 10 mcg/kg epinephrine S.C. stat.
Available: epinephrine 1:1 000 = 1 mg/mL
The child weighs 15 kg.

Step 1:
Calculate the desired dose in mcg (micrograms):
   10 mcg × 15 kg = 150 mcg

Step 2:
   Convert the desired dose to mg:
      1 000 mcg = 1 mg
      150 mcg = N mg
      1 000:1 = 150:N
      1 000 N = 150
$$N = \frac{150}{1\ 000} = 0.15$$
      Answer: give 0.15 mg

Solve:
   Known ratio: 1 mg:1 mL
   Unknown ratio: 0.15 mg:N mL
      1:1 = 0.15:N
      N = 0.15
Answer: give 0.15 mL of epinephrine
Use an accurately calibrated syringe

Exercise 10.1

Complete the following exercise without referring to the previous text. Round all decimal numbers to the nearest hundredth. Correct using the answer guide.

1. A child weighing 17 kg is to receive 5 mg/kg P.O. of an antibiotic. A syrup labeled 25 mg/mL is available.

2. A child weighing 11.5 kg is to receive a stat dose of streptomycin sulfate 20 mg/kg I.M. Medication containing 250 mg/mL is available.

3. The order states: 0.015 mg/kg loading dose of digoxin (Lanoxin). Calculate the dose for a child weighing 4.5 kg if the available strength is 0.25 mg/mL.

4. Is this order safe? The preoperative order for a 10-year-old boy who weighs 34 kg is for atropine sulfate 0.01 mg/kg I.M. 1 hour preoperatively. The literature states that 0.4 mg is the maximum dose that may be given to a child.

5. The order states: Drug A 2 mg/kg P.O. daily in 4 doses. Calculate **each** dose for a patient weighing 5 kg.

6. The infant's weight is 3.9 kg; the order is for Lasix 0.3 mg/kg b.i.d. Lasix 10 mg/mL is available. Calculate the dose to administer.

7. The infant's order is gentamicin 2 mg I.V. q.12h. Gentamicin 20 mg/2 mL is available.

8. The infant's weight is 1 030 g, and the order is for ampicillin 50 mg/kg I.V. q.12h. Ampicillin 250 mg/mL is available.

9. The infant's weight is 860 g, and the order is for morphine 0.09 mg I.V. q.2h. p.r.n. The drug is available in two strengths: 2 mg/mL and 10 mg/mL.

10. The infant weighs 5.3 kg, and the ampicillin order states: 25 mg/kg I.V. in divided doses q.6h. Ampicillin 250 mg/mL is available. Determine the amount of ampicillin in each dose and the number of mL to be given to administer that amount.

Calculations Based on Body Surface Area

Body surface area (B.S.A.) can be used to determine the recommended doses for pediatric patients. B.S.A. is calculated, using a nomogram, on the patient's height and weight. Several such instruments are available. B.S.A. correlates with a number of important physiological factors affecting drug dosage: blood volume, basal metabolic rate, cardiac output, and glomerular filtration.

Calculations for children based on B.S.A. involve two steps: First, calculate the body surface area using a nomogram, as illustrated in Figure 10.1.

Second, calculate the dose to administer using this formula:

$$\frac{child's\ B.S.A.}{1.73\ sq\ m} \times adult\ dose = child's\ dose$$

To calculate B.S.A. using a nomogram, mark the child's height on the left column and weight on the right column, then join these two using a straight edge. The point at which this line crosses the surface area (S.A.) scale gives the B.S.A. in square meters (sq m or m²). For example: a child who is 70 cm tall and weighs 10 kg has B.S.A. of 0.45 m².

Alternatively, if the child is of normal height for weight, the B.S.A. can be based on weight alone using the centre boxed area on the nomogram. Note that the child's weight, expressed in kg in the previous example, is converted to lbs: 10 kg = 22 lbs. Using the centre box you would determine a B.S.A. of 0.46 m², which is very close to the previous calculation.

> Example: Calculate the child's dose of Drug A, if the usual adult dose is 50 mg, and the child's weight is 10 kg and height is 80 cm.
>
> From the nomogram in Figure 10.1, we determine that the child's B.S.A. is 0.48.
>
> Using the formula, calculate the child's dose as follows:
>
> $$\frac{0.48 \, \text{sq m}}{1.73 \, \text{sq m}} \times 50 \, \text{mg} = 13.87 \, \text{mg}$$

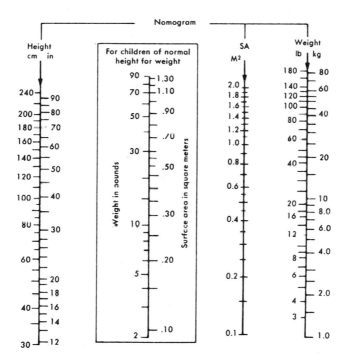

Figure 10.1   Nomogram for calculation of body surface area. (From Behrman, R.E., and Vaughn, V.C., editors: Nelson's textbook of pediatrics, ed. 12, Philadelphia, 1983, W.B. Saunders Co.

Exercise 10.2

Complete the following exercise without referring to the previous text. Round decimal numbers to the nearest hundredth. Correct using the answer guide.

1. The prescriber orders 600 mg/sq m I.V. Calculate the dose for a patient with a B.S.A. of 1.62 sq m.

2. The prescriber orders 30 mg/sq m to be added to 1 L of I.V. fluid. The patient's B.S.A. is 1.58 sq m. Calculate the amount to add if the drug is available in a concentration of 25 mg/mL.

3. A child's B.S.A. is 0.43 sq m. Calculate the recommended dose if the usual adult dose is 150 mg.

4. A child's B.S.A. is 0.29 sq m. Calculate the recommended dose if the usual adult dose is 75 mg.

Use the nomogram in Figure 10.1 to calculate the B.S.A. for each of the following children. Express your answer in hundredths.

5. A child weighing 20 kg with a height of 110 cm.

6. A child weighing 5 kg with a height of 55 cm.

7. A child weighing 13 kg.

8. A child weighing 40 lbs.

9. Recall the discussion in Module 9 on calculating daily fluid replacement. For each of the situations in questions 5 to 8, calculate the daily fluid needs based on this formula:

$$1\ 500\ mL/m^2/day$$

10. For each of the situations in question 9, calculate the rate of flow in ml/hour. Express your answers as whole numbers.

Calculating the Rate of Delivery of I.V. Medications

In some clinical situations, drug dosages are ordered by body weight and by *rate of delivery*. In these situations, several calculations are required. You need to know the dose based on body weight, then determine the *hourly* dose. You must then decide on the amount of drug to add to a specific volume of I.V. fluid. Finally, you must calculate and regulate the rate of flow of the IV. solution, either in mL per hour or drops per minute.

There are several approaches to solving these complex problems. One method is described here:

1. Calculate the required dose, based on the patient's body weight.

2. Calculate the hourly dose required.

3. Determine the amount of drug to add to a specific volume of I.V. fluid. Several factors must be considered, such as stability and compatibility of the drug in the I.V. fluid. These are beyond the scope of this module. If you work in a facility that provides an admixture program, this step will be completed by the pharmacy.

Example:

Mr. J. (weight: 68 kg) is ordered vidarabine monohydrate (Vira-A) 15 mg/kg/daily by constant I.V. infusion. His I.V. is infusing at 100 mL/hour.

Step 1:
Calculate the total daily dose for this patient.

$$15 \times 68 = 1\ 020 \text{ mg/day}$$

Step 2:
Calculate the hourly dose required.

$$\frac{1\ 020}{24} = 42.5 \text{ mg/hour}$$

Step 3:
Determine the amount of drug to add to a specific volume of intravenous fluid.

Let's assume that the drug can be added to 1 L of fluid and infused over 10 hours at the ordered rate of 100 mL/hour. What amount of drug must be added to the L?

The hourly rate is 42.5 mg, and the L will infuse in 10 hours; therefore, $42.5 \times 10 = 425$ mg should be added to the L.

Using the same clinical situation, the following examples are provided to reinforce the steps in this calculation:

Example:

Calculate the amount of Vira-A to be added to a 100-mL minibag and infused over 1 hour.

1. The desired dose is 1 020 mg/day
2. The hourly dose is 42.5 mg/hour.
3. Add 42.5 mg to a 100-mL minibag and infuse over 1 hour.

Example:

Calculate the amount of drug to be added to 500 mL of I.V. fluid and infused at the ordered rate of 100 mL/hr.

1. The desired dose is 1 020 mg/day
2. The hourly dose is 42.5 mg/hour.
3. The 500-mL bag will infuse over 5 hours; therefore, add 5×42.5 mg $= 212.5$ mg to the I.V. bag and infuse over 5 hours at 100 mL/hour.

Critical Care Calculations

Dosages in critical care and emergency units are usually calculated by **titration**, that is, the dose is frequently adjusted to the patient's condition. The dose often will be ordered as a weight or volume of drug per kilogram of body weight per unit of time, for example, 5 mcg/kg/minute.

Drugs used in these settings are potent, and the flow rate must be carefully and accurately monitored. The drugs are delivered by intravenous piggyback (I.V.P.B.), a volutrol or buretrol chamber in the infusion line, and direct I.V. push or bolus. To achieve accuracy, it is safest to use a regulating machine to control the rate of flow and an infusion set that delivers 60 drops/minute (a microdrip set).

Following are two exercises that present opportunities to practice titrating medications. The first focuses on neonates in critical care; the second involves adults in critical care or emergency settings. These calculations require a careful, step-by-step approach. You should write out the problem and the solution, then validate your answer. In many instances, nurses are expected to write the calculations directly on the patient's record and validate their answers with a colleague. Nurses in some settings have devised flow charts or other helpful tools to assist with these calculations, which often vary in response to changes in the patient's parameters. Examples of these tools are also included in this module. See the box on page 122.

Let's use the tool in the box on page 122 to calculate a dopamine drip.

Example:

Infant's weight: 860 g

Order: Dopamine 5 mcg/kg/minute in D-5-W at 1 mL/hour

Solution:

To make 50 mL of solution that provides 5 mcg/kg/minute at a rate of 1 mL/hour:

(5 mcg × 0.86 kg × 60 minutes × 50 mL) = 12 900 mcg dopamine in 50 mL of I.V. solution

View label on page 112 and note the available concentration of dopamine:

40 mg/mL = 40 000 mcg/mL

Calculate the dose of dopamine.

12 900 mcg ÷ 40 000 mcg/mL = 0.32 mL dopamine

Prepare the I.V. solution and run at 1 mL per hour to provide 5 mcg/kg/minute.

Exercise 10.3

Calculate the following problems. Refer to the formula on page 124. For each situation write the problem and the solution, then validate your answers. Round decimal numbers to the nearest hundredth.

1. An infant weighing 600 g is to receive gentamicin sulfate (Garamycin) 2.5 mg/kg I.V. once daily. The drug is supplied in a concentration of 10 mg/mL. Calculate the dose to administer.

    Solution:
    Validation:

2. An infant weighing 1 500 g must receive a loading dose of theophylline elixir of 5 mg/kg orally. This is to be followed by maintenance doses of 1 mg/kg divided into 3 daily doses. The drug is available in a concentration of 80 mg/15 mL. Calculate:

    a. The loading dose
       Solution:
       Validation:
    b. Each maintenance dose
       Solution:
       Validation:

3. An infant's weight is 790 g. The order is for dopamine 5 mcg/kg/minute at 1 mL/hour of D-5-W. Calculate the amount of dopamine to add to a 50 mL I.V. solution. *Do this calculation without any formula, then proceed to the next question.*

    Solution:
    Validation:

4. Use the formula on page 122 to calculate the dosage for question 3.

    _____ mcg dopamine in 50 mL of I.V. solution
    _____ mcg ÷ 40 000 mcg/mL =
    _____ mL dopamine

Your answers for questions 3 and 4 should be the same!

5. For the situation in question 3, calculate the rate of flow in drops per minute using a minidrip set. Use the formula on page 122.

6. For the situation in question 3, refer to the box on page 122.
    a. State the I.V. rate necessary to deliver 2.5 mcg/kg/minute.
    b. Calculate the new rate of flow in drops per minute (minidrip).

7. Refer to the formula on page 122. The infant's weight is 1 170 g. The order is for dopamine 7.5 mcg/kg/minute at 1.5 mL/hour. Calculate:

    a. The required dose of dopamine
       Solution:
       Validation:
    b. The dosage of dopamine received in 1 hour
       Solution:
       Validation:

8. The infant weighs 3.1 kg and is ordered 0.03 mg/kg of atropine sulfate. The available concentration is 0.1 mg/mL. Calculate the dosage.

    Solution:
    Validation:

9. The infant weighs 1 345 g. The order is for lidocaine 1 mg/kg. The available concentration is 20 mg/mL. Calculate the dosage.

    Solution:
    Validation:

10. An isoproterenol drip is running at 1 mL/hour and delivers 0.2 mcg/kg/minute. The infant weighs 1 265 g. How much of the drug does this infant receive each hour?

Titration of Medications

Formula for Mixing Dopamine Solution

To make 50 mL of solution that provides 5 mcg/kg/minute at a rate of 1 ml/hour:

(5 mcg × _____ kg × 60 minutes × 50 mL) = _____ dopamine in 50 mL of I.V. solution

_____ mcg ÷ 40 000 mcg/mL = _____ mL dopamine

Dopamine Drip

Using the solution concentration determined above, the nurse can adjust the I.V. rate in mL/hour as follows:

I.V. Rate	Dopamine Dosage
0.5 mL/hour	2.5 mcg/kg/minute
1 mL/hour	5 mcg/kg/minute
1.5 mL/hour	7.5 mcg/kg/minute

Exercise 10.4

Complete the following exercise by referring to the appropriate figures in the text. *Validate all answers*, then correct using the answer guide.

1. Refer to the box on page 125. For each drug listed, state the total amount of medication contained in the ampule (or vial).

    a. aminophylline
    b. atropine
    c. bretylium (Bretylate)
    d. diazepam (Valium)
    e. dopamine (Intropin)
    f. epinephrine (Adrenalin)
    g. furosemide (Lasix)
    h. isoproterenol HCl (Isuprel)
    i. lidocaine HCl (Xylocaine) ampule
    j. lidocaine HCl (Xylocaine) vial
    k. methoxamine HCl (Vasoxyl)
    l. pancuronium bromide (Pavulon)
    m. procainamide HCl (Pronestyl)
    n. propranolol (Inderal)

2. Prepare an intravenous medication of 250 mg in 250 mL of solution. State the concentration in mcg/mL.

3. Refer to the formula on page 124. Using the solution concentration in the previous question, calculate the rate of flow in drops per minute using a minidrip set to deliver 3.5 mcg/kg/minute for a patient weighing 67 kg.

4. Refer to the box on page 125. Calculate the rate of flow in drops per minute for each of the following patient weights and corresponding medication orders for dopamine:

   a. 65 kg:2 mcg/minute

   b. 70 kg:3 mcg/minute

   c. 69 kg:4 mcg/minute

5. Refer to the box on page 126. The concentration of the epinephrine solution is 4 mcg/mL. State:

   a. The number of mg in 250 mL of I.V. solution

   b. The rate of flow necessary to deliver 2 mcg/minute

   c. How many mcg are delivered in 15 minutes if the rate of flow is 45 drops/minute?

6. Refer to the box on page 126. State:

   a. The concentration of the epinephrine solution in mcg/mL if 4 mg were added to 500 mL

   b. The flow rate required to deliver 1 mcg/minute

   c. How many mcg/minute the patient is receiving if the I.V. pump is set at 23 mL/hour.

Read the case studies, then calculate *all* medications ordered.

> Case Study 1
> Mr. M., age 55, is admitted complaining of chest pain. Telemetry showed short runs of multifocal PVCs followed by ventricular fibrillation. CPR was commenced and I.V. initiated (with a minidrip set). Orders:
>
> lidocaine 100 mg I.V. bolus
> lidocaine commenced 4 mg/minute
> Pronestyl 1 g I.V. bolus
> lidocaine drip discontinued
> Pronestyl drip at 4 mg/minute
> calcium gluconate 1 ampule

Calculate all doses.

7. Lidocaine bolus (see box on page 125).

8. Lidocaine drip; state preparation and flow rate (see boxes on pages 125 and 126).

9. Pronestyl bolus (see box on page 125).

10. Pronestyl drip; state preparation and flow rate (see boxes on pages 125 and 126).

> Case Study 2
> A middle-aged man in the C.C.U. is monitored; he weighs 71 kg. An I.V. is running with a minidrip set and volumetric pump. Respiratory arrest and ventricular tachycardia occur. Orders:
>
> lidocaine 100 mg I.V. bolus
> Valium 5 mg I.V. bolus
> Pavulon 3 mg I.V. bolus
> Xylocaine drip 1 mg/minute
> Lasix 20 mg I.V. bolus
> dopamine drip 3 mcg/kg/minute

Calculate all doses.

11. Lidocaine bolus (see box on page 125).

12. Valium bolus (see box on page 125).

13. Pavulon bolus (see box on page 125).

14. Xylocaine drip; state preparation and flow rate (see boxes on pages 125 and 126).

15. Lasix bolus (see box on page 125).

16. Dopamine drip; state preparation and flow rate. Refer to the box on page 125 to determine the flow rate.

17. Increase the dopamine drip to 4 mcg/kg/minute. Refer to the box on page 125 to determine the flow rate.

> Case Study 3
> Mrs. T. was admitted by ambulance to the C.C.U. She was short of breath and experiencing retro-sternal chest pain radiating to the jaw.
> Orders:
>
> atropine 0.5 mg I.V. bolus
> Isuprel drip 2 mcg/minute

Calculate drug doses.

18. Atropine bolus (see box on page 125).

19. Isuprel drip; state preparation and flow rate (see box on page 126).

20. Increase isoproterenol drip to 2.5 mcg/minute (see box on page 126).

Calculation Formula

To determine flow rate for mcg/kg/minute:

$$\frac{\text{mcg required} \times \text{weight (kg)} \times 60 \text{ minutes/hour}}{\text{mcg per mL}} = \underline{\hspace{1cm}} \text{mL per hour}$$

Example: give dopamine 5 mcg/kg/minute.
Patient weighs 61 kg.

Mix 200 mg in 250 mL:
Concentration = 200 ÷ 250 = 0.8 mg = 800 mcg per mL

$$\frac{5 \text{ mcg} \times 61 \text{ kg} \times 60}{800 \text{ mcg per mL}} = 22.875 \text{ ml/hour}$$

Run at 23 mL/hour = 23 drops per minute (minidrip)

Emergency Medications

Drug	Strength	Volume (ampule or vial)
aminophylline	50 mg/1 mL	10-mL ampule
atropine	0.1 mg/1 mL	10-mL ampule
bretylium (Bretylate)	50 mg/mL	10-mL ampule
diazepam (Valium)	5 mg/mL	2-mL ampule
dopamine (Intropin)	40 mg/mL	5-mL ampule
epinephrine (Adrenalin)	1:1 000 (1 mg/mL)	1-mL ampule
furosemide (Lasix)	10 mg/mL	4-mL ampule
isoproterenol HCl (Isuprel)	1 mg/5 mL	5-mL ampule
lidocaine HCl (Xylocaine)	20 mg/mL	5-mL ampule
lidocaine HCl (Xylocaine)	1 g/50 mL	50-mL vial
methoxamine HCl (Vasoxyl)	20 mg/mL	1-mL ampule
pancuronium bromide (Pavulon)	1 mg/mL	5-mL ampule
procainamide HCl (Pronestyl)	100 mg/mL	5-mL ampule
propranolol (Inderal)	10 mg/mL	1-mL ampule

Dopamine Dosage Table

Add 200 mg to 500 mL solution.

Concentration: 400 mcg/mL solution

Find body weight across the top.
Find desired dose on left side.
Follow line across table to determine flow rate in mL/hour
(or drops per minute using a minidrip set with a drop factor of 60 drops = 1 mL).

mcg/min	Body Weight (in kg)									
	50	55	60	65	70	75	80	85	90	95
1	7	8	9	10	11	11	12	13	13	14
2	15	17	18	19	21	23	24	25	27	29
3	23	25	27	29	31	34	36	38	41	43
4	30	33	36	39	42	45	48	51	54	57
5	37	41	45	49	53	56	60	64	67	71
6	45	49	54	59	63	67	72	77	81	85
7	53	58	63	68	73	79	84	89	95	100
8	60	66	72	78	84	90	96	102	108	113
9	67	74	81	88	95	101	108	115	121	128
10	75	83	90	97	105	113	120	127	135	143

Epinephrine Hydrochloride (Adrenalin) Concentration Table

Prepare the appropriate concentration by mixing the indicated amount of drug in the volume of I.V. solution. Select the dose in mcg per minute in the left column. Follow the line across the table to determine the rate of flow in mL per hour (or drops per minute using a minidrip set with a drop factor of 60 drops = 1 mL).

Dose (mcg/minute)	1 mg/250 mL (4 mcg/mL)	4 mg/500 mL (8 mcg/mL)	2.5 mg/250 mL (10 mcg/mL)
0.5	7	4	—
1	15	8	6
2	30	15	12
3	45	23	18
4	60	30	24
5	75	38	30
6	90	45	36

Lidocaine (Xylocaine) Drip

Add 2 g to 500 mL D-5-W: use a minidrip set (60 drops/mL)

1 mg/minute = 15 mL/hour
2 mg/minute = 30 mL/hour
3 mg/minute = 45 mL/hour
4 mg/minute = 60 mL/hour

Procainamide (Pronestyl) Drip

Add 2 g to 500 mL = 4 mg per mL

1 mg/minute = 15 drops/minute
2 mg/minute = 30 drops/minute
3 mg/minute = 45 drops/minute
4 mg/minute = 60 drops/minute

Isoproterenol HCl (Isuprel) Drip

Add 2 mg to 500 mL I.V. solution = concentration of 4 mcg/mL

1 mcg/minute = 15 drops/minute
2 mcg/minute = 30 drops/minute
3 mcg/minute = 45 drops/minute
4 mcg/minute = 60 drops/minute

POSTTEST

Instructions

1. Write the posttest without referring to any reference materials. Express decimal numbers to the nearest hundredth.

2. Correct the posttest using the answer guide.

3. If your score is 100 percent, congratulations! You have completed the final module.

4. If you don't achieve 100 percent, review the learning package in this module and rewrite the posttest.

1. The drug reference book states that 25 mg/kg of Drug T. is an appropriate dose. The patient weighs 35 kg. Calculate the recommended dosage.

2. Is the following dosage within the recommended guidelines? A child weighing 15 kg is ordered Drug M. 150 mg P.O. The literature suggests 6 to 12 mg/kg of this drug for children.

3. An individual who weighs 70 kg is receiving 250 mg of Drug G. P.O. t.i.d. The recommended dose of this drug is 15 mg/kg/day. Is this patient receiving the recommended dose?

4. Calculate the dose to be administered:
    Ordered: 10 mg/kg P.O.
    Drug available: 200-mg tabs
    Patient weight: 60 kg

5. Calculate the dose to be administered:
    Ordered: 2 mcg/kg I.V. bolus
    Drug available: 400 mcg/mL
    Patient weight: 50 kg

6. Calculate the dose to administer:
    Ordered: 200 mg/sq m
    Drug available: 150 mg/mL
    Patient B.S.A.: 0.91 sq m.

7. If the usual adult dose is 75 mg, calculate the dose for a child whose B.S.A. is 0.29 sq m.

8. If the usual adult dose is 1 g, calculate the dose for a child whose B.S.A. is 0.37 sq m.

9. Order: 30 mg/kg P.O. daily in 3 doses. Patient weighs 65 kg. Calculate each dose.

10. Order: 10 mg/kg I.V. q.6h. Patient weighs 55 kg. Calculate each dose to add to the I.V. if the available strength is 1 g/mL.

Order 1: 2 mcg/kg/minute I.V.

11. For order 1, calculate the dosage required for a patient weighing 63 kg.

12. For order 1, if the I.V. solution contains 1 mg/mL, calculate the rate of flow to deliver the correct dose for a patient weighing 60 kg. The administration set delivers 60 drops/mL.

13. An I.V. is infusing at 15 drops/minute (the drop factor is 60). The concentration of drug is 80 mg in 100 mL I.V. fluid. How much drug in mcg is infusing each minute?

14. If the usual adult dose is 10 mg, calculate the dose for a child with a B.S.A. of 0.2 sq m. The drug is available in 5 mg/mL.

15. Calculate the dose for a patient with a B.S.A. of 1.12 sq m. The order is for 500 mg/sq m, and the drug is available in 250 mg/mL.

A patient on a respirator is ordered gallamine triethiodide (Flaxedil) 1 mg/kg by continuous I.V. infusion. Calculate the dosage for a patient weighing 78 kg, using each of the following available strengths:

16. 1-mL ampule containing 100 mg/mL

17. 10-mL vial containing 20 mg/mL

Order 2: dopamine (Intropin) is ordered at 3 mcg/kg/minute.

18. Using order 2, what is the dose per minute for a patient weighing 79 kg?

19. Using order 2, if the I.V. fluid contains 1 mg/mL of dopamine, calculate the rate of infusion for a patient weighing 79 kg, using a microdrip with a drop factor of 60.

20. Using order 2, calculate the rate of infusion for the same patient, but at a dosage of 3.5 mcg/kg/ minute.

YOUR SCORE: _____ %

100%   YES — you have reached the end of this series of modules. Bravo!
                NO — review this module

Note: if you had any errors on the posttest, analyze your areas of weakness.

Appendix A: Decimal Numbers

Round to the nearest hundredth.

1. $5.6 + 2.3 =$
2. $4.4 + 7.5 =$
3. $6.5 \div 3.2 =$
4. $25.7 \times 2.7 =$
5. $10.6 \times 3.8 =$
6. $8.18 \div 3.12 =$
7. $10.45 \times 2.18 =$
8. $5.72 + 2.85 =$
9. $3.19 + 7.26 =$
10. $10.58 - 3.73 =$

Round to the nearest thousandth.

11. $7.677 \div 2.325 =$
12. $4.294 \div 7.835 =$
13. $10.952 - 2.236 =$
14. $7.735 + 3.257 =$
15. $9.921 \div 10.156 =$
16. $8.652 \times 15.738 =$
17. $9.728 \times 20.327 =$
18. $20.327 \div 10.327 =$
19. $9.777 \div 0.777 =$
20. $15.305 + 8.072 =$

YOUR SCORE: _____ %

Appendix B: Proportion

For each problem, write the proportion equation and solve for N.

1. There are two baskets of fruit with equal ratios of oranges and apples. Basket 1 has 3 oranges and 5 apples. Basket 2 has 9 oranges. How many apples are there in Basket 2?

2. Two classes of children are going on a field trip and want the same ratio of children from grade 2 and 3 in each bus. The first bus has 8 grade two students and 12 grade three students. The second bus has 10 grade two students. How many grade three students should there be in the second bus?

3. A basketball player has a scoring average of 18 of 25 shots. How many baskets will she likely score if she takes 49 shots?

4. The recipe calls for 1 cup of milk and 2 cups of flour. How much milk should be used for 3 cups of flour?

5. A necklace has 5 blue beads to 12 red beads. How many blue beads should there be for 48 red beads?

Write the possible proportion equations for questions 6 and 7.

6. Drug label: 100 mg/2 mL. Give 75 mg.

> Proportion equation #1
> Proportion equation #2
> Proportion equation #3
> Proportion equation #4

7. Drug label: 1 mg/10 mL. Give 0.4 mg.

> Proportion equation #1
> Proportion equation #2
> Proportion equation #3
> Proportion equation #4

Write the proportion equation, solve, and validate.

8. An I.V. fluid has 200 mg in 250 mL. State the concentration in mcg/mL.

> Known ratio:
> Unknown ratio:
> Proportion equation:
> Solution:
> Validation:

9. Vial label states 1 g. Add 4.7 mL of sterile water to yield 5 mL of drug solution. State concentration in mg/mL.

> Known ratio:
> Unknown ratio:
> Proportion equation:
> Solution:
> Validation:

10. Label states 112.5 mg per 5 mL. State as mg/mL.

      Known ratio:
      Unknown ratio:
      Proportion equation:
      Solution:
      Validation:

                YOUR SCORE: _____ %

Appendix C: Dosage Calculations

This appendix provides additional practice in calculating dosages of tablets, liquids, and parenteral medications, reading labels, and reconstituting solutions. The appendix is divided into sections. Select the section you want and answer the questions without referring to the text. Correct using the answer guide.

Section One: Calculating Dosages of Tablets

1. Order: ampicillin 500 mg P.O. b.i.d.
Available: 250-mg tabs
   a. Amount to give?
   b. Number of tabs required per day?
   c. Number of tablets required to give patient for a weekend pass (2 days)?

2. Order: allopurinol (Zyloprim) 300 mg P.O. daily
Available: 100-mg tablets
Amount to give?

3. Order: cephalexin (Keflex) 1 g P.O. q.6h.
Available: 500-mg tablets
Amount to give?

4. Order: levothyroxine sodium (Synthroid) 0.15 mg P.O. daily
Available: 0.05-mg tablets
Amount to give?

5. Order: theophylline (Theo-Dur) 450 mg P.O. p.c.
Available: 300-mg scored tablets
Amount to give?

6. Order: digoxin 125 mcg
Available: 0.125-mg tablets
Amount to give?

7. Order: penicillin G potassium 1 000 000 units q.i.d.
Available: 500 000 units/tablet
Amount to give?

8. Order: ASA 0.65 g P.O.
Available: 325-mg tablets
Amount to give?

9. Order: captopril 0.05 g
Available: 25-mg tablets
Amount to give?

10. Order: sulfadiazine 1.5 g P.O. q.i.d.
Available: 500-mg tablets
Amount to give?

YOUR SCORE: _____ %

Section Two: Calculations of Liquid Preparations

State decimal numbers to the nearest tenth unless otherwise directed.

1. Order: morphine 7.5 mg I.M. p.r.n.
Available: 10 mg/mL
Amount to give (round answer to the nearest hundredth)?

2. Order: NPH insulin 22 units and regular insulin 12 units S.C.
Available: both insulins are concentrated as 100 units/mL
Amount to give (round answer to the nearest hundredth)?

3. Order: hydrocortisone sodium succinate (Solu-Cortef) 75 mg I.M.
Available: 100 mg/2 mL
Amount to give?

4. Order: meperidine (Demerol) 75 mg I.M. stat
Available: 2-mL ampule of 50 mg/mL
Amount to give?

5. Order: fluphenazine (Modecate) 12.5 mg I.M.
Available: 25 mg/mL
Amount to give?

6. Order: heparin 6 000 units
Available: 10 000 units/mL
Amount to give?

7. Order: sodium oxacillin 500 mg I.M.
Available: multidose vial already mixed; label indicates 0.25 g in 1.5 mL
Amount to give?

8. Order: Milk of Magnesia 1 oz
Amount to give in mL?

9. Order: Robitussin 5 to 10 mL p.r.n.
Amount to give in tsp?

10. Order: sodium ampicillin 500 mg I.M. stat
Available: 0.25 g/mL
Amount to give?

YOUR SCORE: _____ %

Section Three: Reading Labels

Refer to the labels on pages 134 and 135 to answer questions 1 to 10.

1. State the concentration of the lidocaine solution, as a percentage and the amount of drug per mL.

2. What is the total amount of lidocaine in the vial?

3. Explain what a 1% solution is.

4. What is the total amount of heparin contained in the multiple-dose vial of heparin sodium injection?

5. How many units of heparin are dissolved in each mL of heparin sodium injection?

6. How much sodium chloride is contained in each mL of heparin sodium injection?

7. Your patient has a heparin lock that must be flushed five times daily with 1 mL of solution. How many days will this box last?

8. How much stronger is the heparin sodium injection than the heparin lock flush solution?

9. What volume of diluent should be added to the Keflin?

10. What is the concentration of the resulting solution in question 9?

YOUR SCORE: _____ %

Section Four: Reconstituting Medications

Refer to the labels below and on page 135 to answer questions 1 to 9.

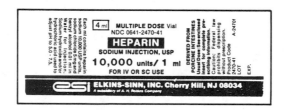

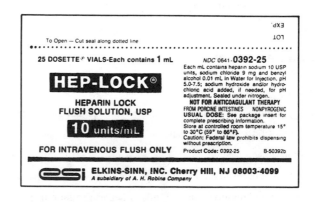

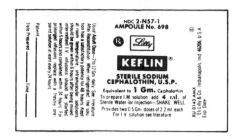

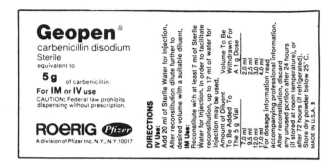

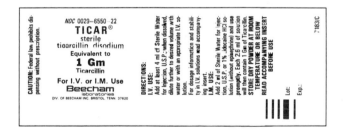

1. Give cephalothin 250 mg I.V. State the procedure for reconstitution and calculate the dosage.

2. Give cephalothin 0.75 g I.V. State the procedure for reconstitution and calculate the dosage.

The label on the Geopen vial indicates that 7 mL of diluent was added today. Calculate the volume required for each of the following patient situations:

3. Give Geopen 1 g I.M.

4. Give carbenicillin disodium 1 500 mg I.M.

5. Refer to the Geopen label. Which procedure produces the most concentrated solution?

    a. Adding 9.5 mL diluent

    b. Adding 17 mL diluent

6. The label on the carbenicillin disodium indicates that 9.5 mL of diluent was added and that 2 mL was given. What dose did the patient receive?

7. Keflin was prepared according to instructions and 1 mL was given. What dose did the patient receive?

8. State the volume of diluent that must be added to ticarcillin disodium for I.V. use.

9. The order is for ticarcillin disodium 1 g I.M. Describe the procedure for reconstitution and calculate the dosage.

10. For the order in question 9, indicate which syringe below shows the correct dosage.

YOUR SCORE: _____ %

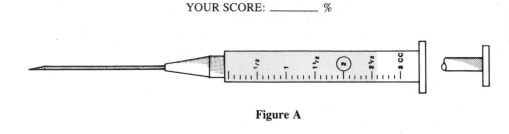

Figure A

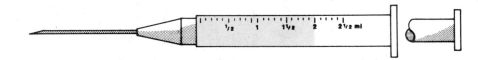

Figure B

Appendix D: Calculating Pediatric Dosages on Body Mass or Age

Clark's Rule

$$\text{Child's dose} = \frac{\text{Mass of child}}{150 \text{ lb or } 68 \text{ kg}} \times \text{Adult dose}$$

Fried's Rule (Birth–12 months)

$$\text{Infant's dose} = \frac{\text{Age (in months)}}{150} \times \text{Adult dose}$$

Young's Rule (1–12 years)

$$\text{Child's dose} = \frac{\text{Age (in yr)}}{\text{Age (in yr)} + 12} \times \text{Adult dose}$$

Appendix E: Sample Examinations for Clinical Instructors

The sample examinations were developed for clinical instructors; consequently no answers are provided. Each examination appears in two formats, one with open questions and an identical examination with a multiple-choice format.

These examinations illustrate a comprehensive test of arithmetic skills with whole numbers, fractions, decimal numbers, use of ratio and proportion, understanding systems of measurement, reading medication labels, and calculating oral and parenteral medications. Nursing students should achieve a perfect score on these examinations or review appropriate sections of the book. The examinations can be used in the clinical setting to assess nursing students' skills before medication administration. The examinations are also useful for periodic reevaluation of students' skills.

Examination 1

1. 57 809 + 3 740 =

2. 6 732 − 599 =

3. 0.76 × 1.95 =

4. 0.25 ÷ 0.125 =

5. 1/3 × 4/9 =

6. 7/15 ÷ 1/2 =

7. Which of the following abbreviations means that a drug is to be administered before meals?
   a. a.c.
   b. p.c.
   c. h.s.

8. How many grams are equivalent to 35 mg?

9. The I.V. order states: infuse 2 000 mL/day. Using a minidrip set (with a drop factor of 60 drops/mL), calculate the rate of flow in mL/hour and drops/minute.

10. How many mL of solution are in the syringe below?

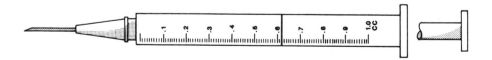

11. The drug is available in 500-mg tablets. How many tablets are required for a dose of 1.5 g?

12. The vial label states NPH insulin 100 units/mL. How many units are contained in 0.4 mL?

13. The order is for 450 000 units of penicillin G and the label states that there are 300 000 units/mL. What amount is required?

14. The label on the penicillin states: 500 000 units/mL. How many units are found in 2.8 mL?

15. The order is for 250 mg of tetracycline. The medication is supplied as a syrup with the concentration of 125 mg/5 mL.
>   a. How many mL are required?
>   b. How many tsp are required?

16. Which of the following tablets provides the smallest amount of medication?
>   a. 0.1 mg
>   b. 0.05 mg
>   c. 0.15 mg

17. The order reads: 75 mg I.M. stat.
Available is a 2-mL ampule with solution concentration of 50 mg/mL.
How many mL should be given?

18. Ordered: Drug New 15 mg P.O. in three divided doses. Available: Drug New 2.5-mg tab.
>   a. State the amount to administer for each dose.
>   b. How many tablets are required for the daily dose?

19. An I.V. that is infusing at 125 mL/hour has been running for 3 hours and 25 minutes. How much solution should have been infused?

20. Two hundred milligrams of a drug is added to 250 mL of I.V. solution. What is the concentration in mcg/mL?

Examination 2

1. 57 809 + 3 740 =
>   a. 61 549
>   b. 62 549
>   c. 61 539

2. 6 732 − 599 =
>   a. 5 133
>   b. 6 133
>   c. 6 123

3. 0.76 × 1.95 =
>   a. 1.482
>   b. 14.82
>   c. 0.148 2

4. 0.25 ÷ 0.125 =
>   a. 5
>   b. 0.5
>   c. 2

5. 1/3 × 4/9 =
>   a. $\dfrac{4}{27}$ b. $\dfrac{9}{12}$ c. $\dfrac{3}{4}$

6. 7/15 ÷ 1/2 =
>   a. $\dfrac{7}{30}$ b. $\dfrac{14}{30}$ c. $\dfrac{14}{15}$

7. Which of the following abbreviations means that a drug is to be administered before meals?

    a. a.c.

    b. p.c.

    c. h.s.

8. How many grams are equivalent to 35 mg?

    a. 0.035

    b. 0.35

    c. 350

9. The I.V. order states: infuse 2 000 mL/day. Using a minidrip set (with a drop factor of 60 drops/mL), calculate the rate of flow in mL/hour.

    a. 33 mL/hour

    b. 83 mL/hour

    c. 125 mL/hour

10. How many mL of solution are in the syringe below?

    a. 0.62

    b. 0.6

    c. 0.64

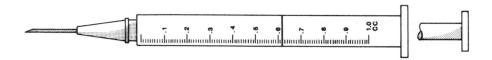

11. The drug is available in 500-mg tablets. How many tablets are required for a dose of 1.5 g?

    a. 3

    b. 2

    c. 2.5

12. The vial label states NPH insulin 100 units/mL. How many units are contained in 0.4 mL?

    a. 4

    b. 40

    c. 400

13. The order is for 450 000 units of pencillin G and the label states that there are 300 000 units/mL. What amount is required?

    a. 1.5 units

    b. 0.67 mL

    c. 1.5 mL

14. The label on the penicillin states: 500 000 units/mL. How many units are found in 2.8 mL?

    a. 1.4 million units

    b. 178 571 units

    c. 140 000 units

15. The order is for 250 mg of tetracycline. The medication is supplied as a syrup with the concentration of 125 mg/5 mL. How many mL are required?

    a. 2 mL

    b. 10 mL

    c. 2.5 mL

16. Which of the following tablets provides the smallest amount of medication?

    a. 0.1 mg

    b. 0.05 mg

    c. 1.15 mg

17. The order reads: 75 mg I.M. stat. Available is a 2-mL ampule with solution concentration of 50 mg/mL. How many mL should be given?

    a. 1.5 mL

    b. 0.67 mL

    c. 3 mL

18. Ordered: Drug New 15 mg P.O. in three divided doses. Available: Drug New 2.5-mg tabs. State the amount to administer for each dose.

    a. 6 tabs

    b. 2 tabs

    c. 7.5 tabs

19. An I.V. that is infusing at 125 mL/hour has been running for 3 hours and 25 minutes. How much solution should have been infused?

    a. 406 mL

    b. 428 mL

    c. 52 mL

20. Two hundred milligrams of a drug is added to 250 mL of I.V. solution. What is the concentration in mcg/mL?

    a. 0.8

    b. 1.25

    c. 800

Examination 3

1. $34\ 989 + 3\ 450 =$

2. $9\ 345 - 209 =$

3. $0.06 \times 4.67 =$

4. $0.05 \div 0.012\ 5 =$

5. $1/6 \times 5/8 =$

6. $5/24 \div 1/3 =$

7. Which abbreviation means that a drug is to be administered at bedtime?

8. How many grams are equivalent to 105 mg?

9. The I.V. order states: infuse 3 000 mL/day. Using a set with a drop factor of 10 drops/mL, calculate rate of flow in:

    a. mL per hour

    b. drops per minute

10. How many mL of solution are in the syringe below?

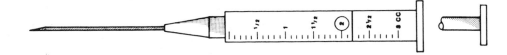

11. The drug is available in 250-mg tablets. How many tablets are required for a dose of 0.5 g?

12. The vial label states: regular insulin 100 units/mL. How many units are contained in 0.34 mL?

13. The order is for 750 000 units of penicillin G; the label states that there are 300 000 units/mL. How many mL are required?

14. The label on the penicillin states: 1 000 000 units/mL. How many units are found in 2.3 mL?

15. The order is for 12.5 mg. The medication is supplied as a syrup with the concentration of 25 mg/5 mL.

    a. How many mL are required?
    b. How many tsp are required?

16. Which of the following tablets provides the largest amount of medication?

    a. 0.1 mg
    b. 0.05 mg
    c. 0.15 mg

17. The order: 45 mg I.M. stat. Available: a 2-mL ampule with solution concentration of 50 mg/mL. How many mL should be given?

18. Ordered: Theo-Dur 900 mg P.O. in 3 divided doses. Available: 300-mg tablets.

    a. What is the amount to administer for each dose?
    b. How many tablets are required for the daily dose?

19. A 1-L bag of I.V. solution is infusing at 75 mL/hour and has been running for 3 hours and 30 minutes.

    a. How much solution should have been infused?
    b. How much solution should remain?

20. Two hundred milligrams of a drug is added to 500 mL of I.V. solution. What is the concentration in mcg/mL?

Examination 4

1. 34 989 + 3 450 =
    a. 38 529
    b. 38 439
    c. 38 349

2. 9 345 − 209 =
    a. 9 136
    b. 9 036
    c. 9 055

3. 0.06 × 4.67 =
    a. 0.028 02
    b. 2.802
    c. 0.280 2

4. 0.05 ÷ 0.012 5 =
    a. 4
    b. 0.4
    c. 0.25

5. 1/6 × 5/8 =

    a. $\dfrac{5}{40}$ b. $\dfrac{5}{48}$ c. $\dfrac{8}{30}$

6. 5/24 ÷ 1/3 =

    a. $\dfrac{5}{6}$ b. $\dfrac{5}{72}$ c. $\dfrac{15}{24}$

7. Which of the following abbreviations means that a drug is to be administered at bedtime?

    a. a.c.
    b. p.c.
    c. h.s.

8. How many grams are equivalent to 105 mg?

    a. 105 000
    b. 0.105
    c. 1.05

9. The IV order states: infuse 3 000 mL/day. Using a set with a drop factor of 10 drops/mL, calculate rate of flow in mL/hour.

    a. 125
    b. 1 250
    c. 21

10. How many mL of solution are in the syringe below?

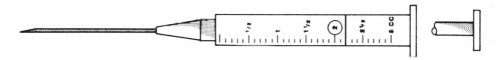

    a. 22 mL
    b. 0.22 mL
    c. 2.2 mL

11. The drug is available in 250-mg tablets. How many tablets are required for a dose of 0.5 g?

    a. 0.5
    b. 2
    c. 5

12. The vial label states: regular insulin 100 units/mL. How many units in 0.34 mL?

    a. 34
    b. 0.34
    c. 3.4

13. The order is for 750 000 units of penicillin G; the label states that there are 300 000 units/mL. How many mL are required?

    a. 2.5 mL
    b. 0.4 mL
    c. 0.25 mL

14. The label on the penicillin states 1 000 000 units/mL. How many units are found in 2.3 mL?

    a. 2 300 000
    b. 230 000
    c. 23 000 000

15. The order is for 12.5 mg. The medication is supplied as a syrup with the concentration of 25 mg/ 5 mL. How many tsp are required?

    a. 2.5
    b. 2
    c. 0.5

16. Which of the following tablets provides the largest amount of medication?

    a. 0.1 mg
    b. 0.05 mg
    c. 0.15 mg

17. The order: 45 mg I.M. stat. Available: a 2-mL ampule with solution concentration of 50 mg/mL. How many mL should be given?

    a. 1.8
    b. 0.9
    c. 1.1

18. Ordered: Theo-Dur 900 mg P.O. in 3 divided doses. Available: 0.3-g tablets. What is the amount to administer for each dose?

    a. 3 tab
    b. 1 tab
    c. 9 tab

19. A 1-L bag of I.V. solution is infusing at 75 mL/hour and has been running for 3 hours and 30 minutes. How much solution should have been infused?

    a. 262.5
    b. 225
    c. 737.5

20. Two hundred milligrams of a drug is added to 500 mL of I.V. solution. What is the concentration in mcg/mL?

    a. 400
    b. 0.4
    c. 2.5

Appendix F: Formulas for Dosage Calculation

Some individuals prefer to learn and use formula to calculate dosages. This is often discouraged because the formula may be forgotten or stated incorrectly. In some situations, the formula will not apply. Consequently, this book has relied on the use of proportion equations. If, however, you do wish to rely on formula, this appendix outlines those for calculating oral and liquid dosages and the rate of I.V. administration.

Calculating dosages of tablets

The oral route is the most common, safest, and economical route of administration. Calculating oral tablets occurs frequently in clinical practice. The formula for this calculation is as follows:

$$\frac{\text{dose desired}}{\text{dose on hand}} = \frac{\text{number of tablets}}{\text{to administer}}$$

Example:

The order is for ascorbic acid 100 mg P.O.
The dose on hand is 50 mg tablets.

$$\frac{\text{dose desired}}{\text{dose on hand}} = \frac{100\,\text{mg}}{50\,\text{mg}} = 2\,\text{tabs}$$

The correct dose to administer is 2 tablets.

When using this formula, the desired dose and the dose on hand *must* be expressed in the same units of measure.

Example:

The order is for 1.5 g of sulfisoxazole (Gantrisin).
Available: 500 mg tablets.
Step 1: convert the order to the same unit of measure as the dose on hand.
    1.5 g = ? mg
    1.5 g = 1 500 mg
Step 2: use the formula

$$\frac{\text{dose desired}}{\text{dose on hand}} = \frac{1\,500\,\text{mg}}{500\,\text{mg}} = 3$$

The correct dose to administer is 3 tablets.

Calculating dosages of liquids

Many medications are administered orally in suspensions and parenterally in solutions. In these situations, the correct dosage to administer is expressed in units of measure of volume (not weight, as in the previous examples). The formula for these calculations is as follows:

$$\frac{\text{dose desired}}{\text{dose on hand}} \times \frac{\text{volume}}{\text{on hand}} = \frac{\text{volume to}}{\text{administer}}$$

The use of the formula is illustrated in the following example. As stated previously, the desired dose and the dose on hand *must* be expressed in the same units of measure.

Example:

The order is thioridazine hydrochloride (Mellaril) 60 mg P.O. On hand is Mellaril 25 mg/5 mL.

$$\frac{\text{dose desired}}{\text{dose on hand}} \times \frac{\text{volume}}{\text{on hand}} = \frac{\text{volume to}}{\text{administer}}$$

$$\frac{60\,\text{mg}}{25\,\text{mg}} \times 5\,\text{mL} = 12\,\text{mL}$$

The correct dosage to administer is 12 mL (which delivers 60 mg of drug).

Calculating rate of flow of intravenous infusions

All intravenous fluids and medications must be administered precisely. The desired rate of flow must be calculated accurately and observed frequently during I.V. therapy. Intravenous fluids are administered either by infusion pump or by gravity drip. When a pump is used the rate of flow is expressed in millilitres per hour. For gravity drip, the rate must be calculated in drops per minute. To calculate the rate of flow, the following formulas can be used.

Example: calculate the rate of flow in mL/hour.

$$\frac{\text{volume of fluid (mL)}}{\text{time to infuse (hours)}} = \text{rate of flow (mL/hour)}$$

The order is: give 3 000 mL of I.V. fluid over 24 hours.

$$\frac{3\,000\,\text{mL}}{24\,\text{hours}} = 125\,\text{mL/hour}$$

Example: calculate the rate of flow in drops/minute.

$$\frac{\text{volume of fluid (mL)}}{\text{time to infuse (minutes)}} \times \frac{\text{calibration of}}{\text{I.V. set}} = \frac{\text{rate}}{\text{of flow}}$$

The order is: give 3 000 mL of I.V. fluid over 24 hours. Use a minidrip set (10 drops/mL)

$$\frac{3\,000\,\text{mL}}{24\,\text{hours} \times 60\,\text{min}} \times 10 = 20.8\,(21\,\text{drops/minute})$$

Answer Guide

Module 1

Arithmetic of Whole Numbers

1. 1 223
2. 2 517
3. 814
4. 594
5. 475
6. 1 354
7. 53
8. 789
9. 51 684
10. 8 385
11. 890 415
12. 2 189 094
13. 5
14. 8
15. 5
16. 8

Arithmetic of Fractions

1. $\dfrac{34}{39}$

2. $\dfrac{101}{112}$

3. $\dfrac{23}{30}$

4. $1\dfrac{5}{12}$

5. $\dfrac{7}{16}$

6. $\dfrac{1}{4}$

7. $\dfrac{7}{24}$

8. $\dfrac{1}{24}$

9. $28\dfrac{31}{56}$

10. $1\dfrac{5}{12}$

11. $7\dfrac{29}{64}$

12. $8\dfrac{1}{3}$

13. $1\dfrac{11}{24}$

14. $\dfrac{3}{4}$

15. $9\dfrac{3}{4}$

16. $\dfrac{50}{63}$

17. $3\dfrac{3}{7}$

18. 12

19. $\dfrac{1}{4}$

20. b

21. $\dfrac{1}{4} = \dfrac{4}{16}$

Arithmetic of Decimal Numbers

1. 0.5
2. 5.7
3. 5.61
4. 5 792.178
5. 314.488
6. 22.283 1
7. 3.7
8. 0.875
9. 0.9
10. $\dfrac{75}{100}$ $\dfrac{3}{4}$
11. 1.01   0.1   0.01   0.001
12. $\dfrac{1}{4}$
13. 0.25
14. 25%
15. $\dfrac{5}{6}$
16. 0.83
17. 83%
18. $\dfrac{1}{1\,000}$
19. 0.001
20. 0.1%

Word Problems

1. 76%
2. $5.00
3. 30
4. 7
5. $20
6. $10
7. a. $450.00
   b. 41%
8. a. $\frac{42}{50}$ or $\frac{21}{25}$ will be seated

   b. $\frac{8}{50}$ or $\frac{4}{25}$ must stand

   c. 16%
9. $6.50
10. $262
11. $3
12. 3
13. 16 sticks of licorice and $0.40 change
14. 13 822
15. $12.50
16. 5
17. $2.25
18. 11 days
19. $130.15

Systems of Measurement and Abbreviations

1. 10 000
2. 0.05
3. 250
4. 1 250
5. 1 000
6. 2 000
7. 0.35
8. 150
9. 700 000
10. 102
11. 10
12. 77
13. 65
14. after meals
15. as necessary
16. immediately
17. tablet
18. twice a day
19. at bedtime
20. ointment
21. milligram
22. microgram

23. subcutaneous
24. milliequivalent
25. before meals

Dosage Calculations

1. 2
2. 2
3. b
4. 1 tablet three times a day and 4 tablets at bedtime
5.

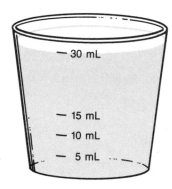

6. ⎱
7. ⎰ See opposite page
8. 1 mL
9. 100
10. 120
11. 31
12. 21
13. 25
14. a. 125
    b. 42
15. 0.4 mL
16. 0.7 mL
17. a
18. 250 000
19. 75 mcg (0.075 mg)
20. Choices: a. give 5 tabs of 0.025-mg strength
             b. give 1 tabs of 0.05-mg strength and 1 tab of 0.075-mg strength
             c. or give 2 tabs of 0.05-mg strength and 1 tab of 0.025-mg strength
    Validation: 0.05
                0.05
                $\underline{0.025}$
                0.125 mg

6.

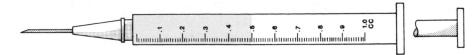

7.

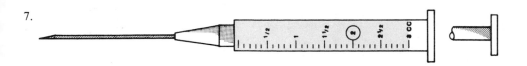

Module 2

Pretest

1. $3\dfrac{13}{20}$

2. $1\dfrac{7}{30}$

3. $2\dfrac{3}{4}$

4. $7\dfrac{7}{24}$

5. $1\dfrac{11}{21}$

6. $\dfrac{31}{32}$

7. $\dfrac{15}{16}$

8. $\dfrac{47}{72}$

9. $\dfrac{13}{20}$

10. $2\dfrac{9}{16}$

11. $2\dfrac{15}{16}$

12. $\dfrac{5}{28}$

13. $\dfrac{17}{144}$

14. $\dfrac{1}{40}$

15. $\dfrac{1}{2}$

16. $14\dfrac{5}{8}$

17. $4\dfrac{4}{5}$

18. $31\dfrac{1}{2}$

19. $1\dfrac{1}{4}$

20. $\dfrac{3}{16}$

21. $5\dfrac{1}{8}$

22. $\dfrac{8}{9}$

23. 3

24. $101\dfrac{1}{3}$

25. $\dfrac{3}{16}$

26. $133\dfrac{1}{3}$

27. 22

28. $1\dfrac{1}{48}$

29. $3\dfrac{3}{5}$

30. $7\dfrac{6}{11}$

31. $8\dfrac{1}{6}$

32. $3\dfrac{25}{34}$

33. $4\dfrac{7}{8}$

34. $10\dfrac{5}{12}$

35. 4

36. 30

37. 40

38. 24
39. $\frac{7}{8}$
40. $\frac{1}{4}$
41. $\frac{2}{3}$
42. $\frac{3}{7}$
43. $\frac{5}{8}$
44. $\frac{1}{15}$
45. Proper fraction
46. Improper fraction
47. Mixed number
48. Proper fraction··
49. Proper fraction
50. Proper fraction
51. Mixed number
52. Improper fraction
53. $\frac{3}{6}$
54. $\frac{9}{60}$
55. $\frac{21}{27}$
56. $\frac{49}{70}$
57. $\frac{6}{30}$
58. No
59. Yes
60. $\frac{49}{8}$
61. $\frac{79}{10}$
62. $\frac{11}{2}$
63. 9
64. $\frac{4}{8}$ or $\frac{1}{2}$
65. 32
66. $\frac{1}{8}$
67. $\frac{2}{5} \times 30 = 12$ ounces·
68. $1\frac{11}{20}$ cups

Posttest

1. $\frac{25}{28}$
2. $1\frac{21}{40}$
3. $\frac{13}{14}$
4. $14\frac{7}{12}$
5. $\frac{37}{60}$
6. $1\frac{7}{18}$
7. $\frac{17}{36}$
8. $2\frac{1}{3}$
9. $1\frac{1}{5}$
10. $20\frac{1}{16}$
11. $\frac{5}{24}$
12. $\frac{43}{120}$
13. $\frac{2}{21}$
14. $\frac{3}{5}$
15. 75
16. $7\frac{2}{3}$
17. 3
18. 78
19. $\frac{3}{4}$
20. $9\frac{3}{4}$
21. $\frac{9}{10}$
22. $\frac{5}{12}$
23. $\frac{50}{63}$
24. $13\frac{1}{3}$
25. $\frac{38}{3}$

26. $\frac{14}{4}$

27. $4\frac{1}{5}$

28. $4\frac{2}{9}$

29. $2\frac{3}{4}$

30. $12\frac{5}{7}$

31. $16\frac{11}{12}$

32. $3\frac{1}{3}$

33. 72
34. 48
35. 72
36. 42

37. $\frac{4}{9}$

38. $\frac{5}{9}$

39. $\frac{5}{6}$

40. 3

41. $\frac{8}{9}$

42. $\frac{14}{11}$

43. $1\frac{2}{3}$

44. $\frac{35}{49}$

45. $\frac{28}{70}$

46. $\frac{60}{108}$

47. $\frac{30}{200}$

48. $\frac{32}{44}$

49. 17
50. 80
51. 20 minutes

52. 40

53. No; the correct answer is $1\frac{1}{5}$

54. $\frac{1}{5}$

Module 3

Pretest

1. 0.25
2. 1
3. 0.12
4. 3.4
5. 7.1
6. 1.2
7. 9.2
8. 12.46
9. 6.1
10. 34
11. 4.91
12. 2.547
13. 126.034 2
14. 6.27
15. 3.732
16. 6.3
17. 3.3
18. 4.52
19. 0.05
20. 8
21. 80
22. 800
23. 0.001
24. 0.5
25. 66.66 (repeating)
26. 2.2233 (repeating)
27. 44.5
28. 0.8
29. 0.5
30. 0.3
31. 0.8
32. $\frac{3}{5}$ or $\frac{6}{10}$

33. $\frac{57}{100}$

34. $1\frac{1}{4}$

35. $\frac{1}{100}$

36. 0.000 1   0.01   0.1   1.001   1.101
37. $1.20
38. $11.70
39. $95.40
40. $11.37

Exercise 3.1

1. Correct
2. 1.7
3. Correct
4. 0.35
5. 1.4
6. 1.9
7. 1
8. 1.1
9. 6.33
10. 2.09
11. 0.95
12. 7.67
13. 1.055   1.105   1.15   1.515
14. 50.6   5.06   0.506

Exercise 3.2

1. 6.44
2. 14.373
3. 11.21
4. 1.76
5. 2.046 1
6. 40 074.820 7

Exercise 3.3

1. 4.064
2. 3.822
3. 3.426 52
4. 58.143 06
5. 4.3
6. 879.4
7. 0.5
8. 1 000 250

Exercise 3.4

1. $\frac{1}{8}$
2. $2\frac{1}{2}$
3. $\frac{3}{5}$
4. $\frac{3}{4}$
5. $1\frac{3}{4}$

6. 0.75
7. 0.05
8. 3.83 (repeating)
9. 0.33 (repeating)
10. 1.25

Exercise 3.5

1. 150%
2. 37%
3. 17%
4. 94%
5. 6.66% (repeating)
6. 83.33% (repeating)
7. 72.72% (repeating)
8. 79%
9. 0.77
10. 0.01
11. 0.29
12. 0.82
13. $\frac{1}{4}$
14. $\frac{33}{100}$
15. $\frac{3}{50}$
16. $\frac{12.5}{100} = \frac{125}{1\ 000} = \frac{1}{8}$

Posttest

1. 4.15
2. 1.77
3. 1.26
4. 1.32
5. 2.33
6. 1.89
7. 1.19
8. 2.42
9. 10.63
10. 0.3
11. 4.25
12. 101
13. 180
14. 0.13
15. 2
16. 3
17. 4.2
18. 1.8
19. 1.3

20. 2.3
21. 1.89
22. 1.97
23. 10.64
24. 0.36
25. 0.67
26. 1.25
27. 0.88
28. 2.5
29. $\frac{19}{25}$
30. $1\frac{3}{10}$
31. $\frac{13}{100}$
32. $\frac{1}{20}$
33. 0.5
34. 1.2
35. 1.01
36. 1.901, 1.991, 10.01, 10.1
37. $451.08
38. $386.77
39. $3.92
40. $527.14

Module 4

Pretest

1. 45
2. 12
3. 25
4. 4
5. 4
6. 3
7. $\frac{1}{100}$
8. 0.01
9. 1%
10. $\frac{1}{5}$
11. 0.2
12. 20%
13. $\frac{1}{250}$
14. 0.004
15. 0.4%

16. 0.5
17. 165
18. 2 000
19. 12.5
20. 7:5
21. 5:1
22. 17:3
23. 1.5
24. A relationship that exists between two quantities
25. An equation between two equal ratios

Exercise 4.1

1. 1:9
2. 9:10
3. 325 units per tab or 325:1
4. 25 units per tsp or 25:1
5. 1:4

Exercise 4.2

1. $\frac{1}{25}$
2. 0.04
3. 4%
4. $\frac{1}{10}$
5. 0.1
6. 10%
7. $\frac{7}{9}$
8. 0.8
9. 77.8%
10. $\frac{25}{2}$
11. 12.5
12. 1 250%
13. $\frac{50}{1}$
14. 50
15. 5 000%
16. $\frac{10}{1}$
17. 10
18. 1 000%
19. 3:4
20. 333:1 000
21. 1:2
22. 1:200

Exercise 4.3

1. 8
2. 25
3. 21
4. 2
5. 1.5
6. 1.33 (repeating)
7. 0.37
8. 0.5
9. 0.25
10. 1
11. 4
12. 1 080
13. 1
14. 0.5
15. $N = \dfrac{3}{5}$
16. 4 scoops:6 cups = N scoops:24 cups

    4:6 = N:24

    6 N = 4 × 24 × 96

    $N = \dfrac{96}{6}$

    N = 16

    Answer: use 16 scoops

    Validate: 4:6 = 16:24

17. 1 cup milk:1.5 cups mix = N cups milk:4 cups mix

    1.5 N = 4

    N = 2.66

    Answer: use 2.66 (or 2.7 or $2\frac{2}{3}$) cups of milk

18. 1 pkg gum:3 pkgs mints = N gum:45 mints

    1:3 = N:45

    3 N = 45

    N = 15

    Answer: you need 15 pkgs of gum

19. 22 children:33 hot dogs = 28 children:N hot dogs

    22:33 = 28:N

    22 N = 924

    N = 42

    Answer: you cook 42 hot dogs

20. 1 cup lime juice:3 cups apple juice = N cups lime juice: 20 apple juice

    1:3 = N:20

    3 N:20

    N = 666

    Answer: 6.7 or $6\frac{2}{3}$ cups of lime juice

Posttest

1. 9
2. 8
3. 10
4. 23:39
5. 3:17
6. A relationship that exists between two quantities
7. An equation between two equal ratios
8. 7
9. 10 units/tsp or 10:1
10. No; the two ratios are not equal. Validate by multiplication; multiply means and extremes.

    6:32 = 24:100

    6 × 100 = 600

    32 × 24 = 768
11. $\dfrac{0.9}{100}$ or 9:1 000
12. $\dfrac{1}{1}$
13. 1
14. 100%
15. $\dfrac{2}{3}$
16. 0.7
17. 66.7%
18. $\dfrac{1}{1\ 000}$
19. 0.001
20. 0.1%
21. $\dfrac{3}{250}$
22. $\dfrac{4}{125}$
23. $\dfrac{1}{8}$
24. $\dfrac{2}{5}$
25. 1 red:8 green = 12 red:N green
26. 1:8 = 12:N

    N = 8 × 12 = 96

    Answer: 96 green beads
27. Validation: 1:8 = 12:96

    96 = 96
28. 2 tablespoons:3 cups = N tablespoons:8 cups
29. 2:3 = N:8

    3 N = 16

    $N = \dfrac{16}{3} = 5\frac{1}{3}$ tablespoons

30. Validation: $2:3 = 5\frac{1}{3}:8$

    $16 = 16$

Module 5

Pretest

1. metre, m
2. kilogram, kg
3. mole, mol
4. 0.1
5. 0.01
6. 0.001
7. 0.000 000 001
8. 0.000 001
9. 1 000
10. 1 000 mg
11. 1 000 mL
12. 0.01 g
13. 1 000 g
14. 0.001 g
15. 0.25 L
16. 0.04 kg
17. 0.2 g
18. 300 mg
19. 100 cm
20. 2.5 m
21. 600 mg
22. 60 mL
23. 5 mL
24. 6.6 lb
25. 182.88 cm

Exercise 5.1

1. k
2. d
3. c
4. m
5. mc or μ
6. 1 000
7. 0.000 000 001
8. 0.000 000 000 001
9. 0.001
10. 0.000 001

11. 0.01
12. kilo, hecto, deci, centi, milli, micro, nano, pico

Exercise 5.2

1. m
2. 10 kg
3. 0.5 mL
4. L
5. 1 000 mL
6. 51 517
7. True

Exercise 5.3

1. 1 000
2. 1 000
3. 100
4. 1
5. 1 000 000
6. 0.25
7. 500
8. 200
9. 1.000
10. 0.001
11. 0.3
12. 0.8
13. 1.5
14. 750
15. 2.5

Exercise 5.4

1. 79.54
2. 79.5
3. 80
4. 55
5. 4 feet 7 inches
6. 5
7. 30

Posttest

1. 2 000
2. 0.25
3. 2

4. 6 000
5. 7 000
6. 5
7. 0.001 25
8. 3
9. 2 500
10. 500
11. 1.456
12. 0.000 5
13. 1 000
14. 170
15. 1.79
16. 500
17. 0.25
18. 1 340
19. 10 000 000
20. 79 000 000
21. 0.01
22. 0.001
23. 0.000 001
24. 1 000
25. 0.1

Module 6

Pretest

1. Morphine sulfate 10 to 15 mg intramuscularly every 4 hours as necessary
2. Insulin 6 units subcutaneously immediately
3. Metoclopramide 10 mg by mouth, before meals, three times a day
4. Aluminum hydroxide 30 mL by mouth, 1 hour after meals, three times a day
5. Flurazepam hydrochloride 15 mg by mouth at bedtime
6. tablet
7. solution (or liquid)
8. 5 mg/tablet
9. 10 mg/mL
10. Dosage
11. Route
12. False: it contains slightly more than 1 mL to allow extra fluid to fill the needle
13. E
14. G
15. F
16. C

17. H
18. I
19. B
20. A
21. D
22. J
23. 75 mL,
    33 mL,
    11.5 mL
24. 20 million u
25. 500 000 u/mL
26. penicillin G potassium
27. Pfizerpen
28. I.V.
29. 6 to 40 million u
30. the twenty-second day of the month
31. A substance dissolved in a solvent
32. A homogeneous mixture containing one or more dissolved substances in a liquid
33. The liquid in which another substance is dissolved
34. Is determined by the amount of solute dissolved in a given amount of solvent

Exercise 6.1

1. Meperidine 50 to 75 mg intramuscularly every 3 to 4 hours as necessary
2. Acetaminophen 650 mg by mouth every 4 hours
3. Codeine 60 mg by mouth immediately and every 4 hours
4. Penicillin 500 000 units intravenously four times a day
5. Phenobarbital elixir 100 mg at bedtime
6. Patient
7. Drug
8. Dosage or dose
9. Route
10. Frequency or time of administration

Exercise 6.2

1. tablet
2. 325 mg/tab
3. Acetaminophen
4. Colace
5. Docusate sodium
6. 1 to 3 Tbsp; 15 to 45 mL

7. Liquid
8. 20 mg/5 mL
9. 240 mL (8 × 30)
10. 24 days

Exercise 6.3

1. Solution
2. Solute
3. Solvent
4. Penicillin G potassium
5. Sterile water
6. True
7. b
8. a
9. g
10. mL
11. mL
12. mL
13. weight per volume (w/v)
14. volume per volume (v/v)

Posttest

Part One: crossword

Across	Down
1. PRN	1. PO
3. Q4H	2. UNG
5. STAT	3. QID
8. PC	4. HS
10. BID	6. TID
12. AC	7. TAB
13. QS	9. CAPS
	11. IM
	13. QH

Part two

1. Solution
2. 1 mL
3. 10 mg/mL
4. 25 vials
5. Protect from light
6. Yes
7. Every 3 hours if necessary
8. Prepare as directed; slight discoloration does not alter drug effect

9. Digoxin 250 micrograms orally daily
10. Indocid 50 milligrams orally three times a day
11. Phenobarbital 25 milligrams orally at bedtime
12. Benadryl 25 milligrams orally four times a day
13. Pro-Banthine 15 milligrams orally before meals and 30 milligrams at bedtime
14. Demerol 75 milligrams intramuscularly every 3 to 4 hours as required
15. Amikacin 15 milligrams per kilogram intravenously per day
16. A substance dissolved in a solvent
17. A homogeneous mixture that contains one or more dissolved substances in a liquid
18. The liquid in which another substance is dissolved
19. Is determined by the amount of solute dissolved in a given amount of solvent
20. 100 parts

Module 7

Pretest

1. 3 tablets
2. 2 tablets
3. 2 tablets
4. 1.5 tablets
5. 2 tablets
6. 0.5 tablet
7. 3 tablets
8. 0.5 tablet
9. 168 capsules
10. 1 tablet of 125 mcg strength daily
11. 1 tablet of phenobarbital 15-mg strength twice daily
12. 1 tablet of baclofen 10-mg strength three times daily
13. 2 softgels at bedtime
14. 1 tablet 15-mg strength in a.m. and 1 tab 30 mg at bedtime
15. 1 tablet 250-mcg (or 0.25-mg) strength daily
16. 250 mcg
17. 1 30-mg tablet and 1 15-mg tablet strength of phenobarbital

18. Give $\frac{1}{2}$ tablet of 10-mg strength three times a day for 4 days, then 1 tablet of 10-mg strength three times a day for 3 days; total number of tablets: 15
19. 300 mg
20. 1 tablet 30-mg strength two times daily and 1 tablet 30 mg plus 1 tablet 15-mg strength at bedtime; total daily dose is 105 mg

Exercise 7.1

1. 2 tablets
2. 3 tablets (1.5 g = 1 500 mg)
3. 2 tablets (0.2 g = 200 mg)
4. $1\frac{1}{2}$ tablets (1.5 tablets)
5. 2 tablets
6. Either six of the 5-mg tablets or one of the 20-mg tablets and two of the 5-mg tablets
7. $\frac{1}{2}$ tablet (0.5 tablet)
8. 2 tablets
9. $\frac{1}{2}$ tablet (0.5 tablet)
10. 2 capsules (0.5 g = 500 mg)

Exercise 7.2

1. 473 mL
2. 200 mL
3. 480 mL
4. 120 mL
5. 237 mL on label (240 mL approximately = 8 × 30)
6. 5 mL
7. 1 tsp.
8. 10 mL
9. 4 mL
10. 1 tsp.
11. 7.5 mL
12. 2.5 mL
13. 4 mL
14. 1 tsp.
15. 1 mL
16. approximately 47 doses (5 mL per dose)
17. 6 doses (20 mL per dose)
18. 40 doses (5 mL per dose)
19. 473 doses (1 mL per dose)
20. 64 doses (7.5 mL per dose

Posttest

1. 3 tablets
2. 1.5 tablets
3. 2 tablets
4. 2 tablets
5. 2 tablets
6. 14 tablets
7. 2 tablets
8. 1.5 tablets
9. 5 mL
10. 1.25 = 1.3 mL
11. 3.75 = 3.8 mL
12. 200 mg (if teaspoon is standard size)
13. 1.875 = 1.9 mL
14. 0.5 tablet
15. 4 mL
16. 1 600 units = 1 mg (200 000 units = 125 mg)
17. 3.125 = 3.1 mL
18. 375 mcg
19. 18 920 mg (200 mg/5 mL)
20. 40 000 units/mL

Module 8

Pretest

1. 0.8 mL
2. 0.4 mL
3. 0.22 mL
4. 0.12 mL
5. 0.34 mL
6. 0.7 mL
7. 1.5 mL
8. 0.75 mL
9. Incorrect; should be 0.5 mL; include zero before decimal
10. Incorrect; should be 1 mL; an ampule contains slightly more than 1 mL
11. Incorrect calculation; correct answer is 0.5 mL
12. No: should be 4.3 mL
13. 0.6 mL
14. Add 1 mL of water, mix thoroughly, then give entire amount, which will be slightly more than 1 mL
15. 1 g/mL
16. 1.5 mL

17. 3 mL
18. Give 1 mL of morphine 10-mg/mL strength
19. Give 0.75 mL of morphine 10-mg/mL
strength, or give 0.5 mL of morphine-15 mg/
mL-strength
20. 0.75 mL
21. Use 0.8 mL of morphine 15-mg/mL
strength
22. 6 mg
23. 2.5 mL
24. 5.7 mL
25. 3.5 mL
26. 330 mg/mL
27. 250 mg/1.5 mL
28. 250 mg/mL
29. 1.52 mL
30. 1.8 mL

Exercise 8.1

1. 0.75 mL
2. 75 mg
3. 1.6 mL
4. 1.5 mL
5. 2 mL
6.

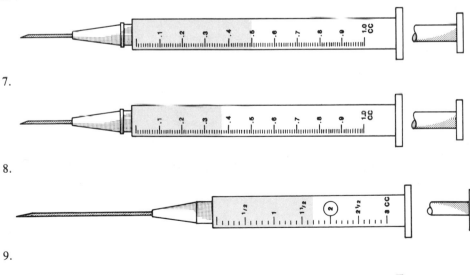

7.

8.

9.

10.

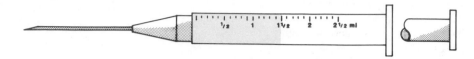

Exercise 8.2

1. Add 9.3 mL
2. Give 1.33 mL
3. 3.75 mL
4. 2 mL
5. 1.25 mL
6. 250 000 units
7. 200 000 units
8. 350 000 units
9. Add 1.6 mL diluent; give 2 mL
10. Add 4.6 mL diluent; give 2 mL
11. Give 1.5 mL
12. On the fourteenth day of the month
13. Add 5.7 mL diluent; give 2 mL
14. Add 5.7 mL diluent; give 1.5 mL
15. On the twenty-fifth day

Posttest

1. 1.33 mL
2. 3
3. 0.25 mL
4. 0.35 mL
5. 0.15 mL
6. 0.5 mL
7. Yes (0.22 + 0.08 = 0.3)
8. Give 1.2 mL; add 1.6 mL
9. 0.8 mL
10. 1 mL
11. 1.8 mL
12. 2.5 mL
13. 100 000 units/mL
14. 2.5 mL
15. At 1300 hours on the twenty-fourth day of the month
16. 1 mL; 10 mg/100 mL = 1 mg/10 mL
17. 7 days
18. 24 hours at room temperature 4 days in refrigerator
19. I.M., I.V.
20. I.M., I.V.
21. 1 million units

22. 4 g
23. Total: 0.36 mL
24. 0.75 mL
25. Add 5.7 mL of diluent; give 2 mL
26. 1 000 000/mL
27. 0.5 mL
28. 20 doses
29. 500 units
30. 3 700 units

Module 9

Pretest

1. Approximately 2 mL/minute
2. Approximately 21 drops per minute
3. 20
4. 83 mL/hour
5. Approximately 83 drops per minute
6. 25 drops per minute
7. 83 mL/hour
8. Approximately 83 drops per minute
9. 10 drops per minute
10. 563 mL
11. 50 drops per minute
12. No, should be approximately 17 drops per minute
13. 8
14. 42 drops per minute
15. 2 hours
16. 100 drops per minute
17. 33 drops per minute
18. 25 mL infused = 250 mg of drug infused
19. Add 2 mL to 25 mL = 27 mL run over 10 minutes
    Run at 54 drops per minute
    Add 2 mL to 25 mL = 27 mL over 15 minutes
    Run at 36 drops per minute
20. 50 drops/minute

Exercise 9.1

1. Approximately 83 drops per minute
2. 20
3. Approximately 21 drops
4. Approximately 125 drops per minute
5. 100 mL/hour
6. 3 600 mL
7. 150 hour
8. 25 drops per minute
9. 167 drops per minute
10. 42 drops per minute

Exercise 9.2

1. 209 lbs = 95 kg; first 10 kg give 100 ×
10 = 1 000 mL;
next 10 kg give 50 mL × 10 = 500 mL;
remaining 75 kg give 20 mL/kg = 75 × 20 =
1 500 mL;
total = 3 000 mL
2. 42 lbs = 19 kg; first 10 kg give 100 mL/kg =
100 × 10 = 1 000 mL
next 9 kg give 50 mL/kg = 50 × 9 = 450 mL;
total = 1 450 mL
3. 12 lbs 402 = 5.57 kg × 100 mL/kg = 557
mL
4. Total fluid needs:2 100mL in 24 hours
5. Total fluid needs: 2 240 mL in 24 hours
6. 3 000 mL = 150 g dextrose = 1 695
kilojoules
7. 1 450 mL = 72.5 g dextrose = 819
kilojoules
8. 557 mL = 27.85 g dextrose = 314.7
kilojoules
9. 2 100 mL = 105 g dextrose = 1 187
kilojoules
10. 2 240 mL = 112 g dextrose = 1 266
kilojoules

Exercise 9.3

1. a. 80 drops per minute
   b. 3.3 mg/minute
2. a. 100 drops per minute
   b. 8.3 mg/minute
3. new volume = 120 mL; 120 drops per
minute
4. 150 drops per minute
5. a. 42 drops per minute
   b. 125 mL:60 minutes = 100 mL:N; 48
   minutes

6. a. 0.4 mL
   b. 100 mL over 4 hours = 25 drops per
   minute
7. a. 1.75 mL (or 1.8 mL)
   b. 50 drops per minute
8. a. 125 drops per minute
   b. 0.8 mL
   c. 24 minutes 1324 hours
9. a. Add 4 mL sterile water; shake well
   b. 2.2 mL
   c. Add to 75 mL and infuse at 19 drops per
   minute
10. a. Two doses
    b. 33 drops per minute
11. a. Add 8.6 mL sterile water
    b. 2 mL
    c. 100 drops per minute
12. methicillin sodium (Staphcillin)
    cefazolin sodium (Ancef)
    sodium cephalothin (Keflin)
13. 4 mL
14. 4 mL
15. 5 mL

Posttest

1. Approximately 125 drops per minute
2. Approximately 21 drops per minute
3. Volume required is 100 L of I.V. fluid;
dilute 100 mg of the drug in 100 mL of I.V.
fluid; infuse over 2 hours = 50 mL, therefore
50 mg per hour
4. 50 drops per minute
5. 25 mg of aminophylline
6. 10 hours; 500 mg of drug added to 500 mL
of I.V. fluid to provide a concentration of 1 mg/
mL; infuse at 50 mg (therefore 50 mL) per hour
7. 50 mL of I.V. fluid; add 250 mg of the drug
to 50 mL of the I.V. fluid to provide a
concentration of 5 mg/mL
8. 100 drops per minute
9. 375 mL should have been absorbed in 3
hours; the I.V. is 75 mL behind
10. The new rate of flow is 23 drops per minute
11. 28 drops per minute
12. 60 minutes or 1 hour
13. 1200 hours
14. 1 500 mL
15. 480 mL

16. a. Add 19 mL of diluent; withdraw 10 mL for 1 dose
    b. 125 mL/hour = 42 drops per minute
    c. Add 10 mL of the drug solution to 53 mL of the I.V. solution = 63 mL I.V. solution to infuse over 30 minutes
17. a. Dilute with 20 mL and use entire contents of vial for loading dose
    b. 17 drops per minute
    c. 126 g of sodium
    d. Add 20 mL of the drug solution to 80 mL of the I.V. solution and infuse over 1 hour
18. a. 125 drops per minute
    b. 0.5 mL
    c. 1 L
    d. 5 000 units in 8 hours (or 480 minutes) = N units/minute
       5 000/480:N/1
       480 N = 5 000
       N = 10.42
       Approximately 10 units/minute
19. a. 100 mL of I.V. solution containing 250 mg of the drug
    b. 33 drops per minute
20. a. 125 drops per minute
    b. 100 drops per minute
    c. 3 000mg (or 3 g)
    d. Drug doses are administered 6 times for 30 minutes each time at a rate of 50 mL over 30 minutes; total volume of medication solution = 3 hours × 100 mL/hour = 300 mL of solution with medication. I.V. infusing at 125 mL/ hour for remaining 21 hours = 125 × 21 = 2 625 mL. Total: 300 + 2 625 = 2 925 mL.

Module 10

Pretest

1. 0.1 mL
2. 0.9g (or 900 mg)
3. 6.9 mg
4. 144.5 mg
5. 24.9 mg
6. 800 mcg/mL
7. 15 drops per minute

8. 4 mg/mL
9. Approximately 16 drops per minute
10. 130 mcg/minute
11. 800 mcg/mL
12. Approximately 10 drops per minute
13. 4 mcg/mL
14. 6.5 mg
15. 200 mcg or 0.2 mg per minute
16. a. 3 mL
    b. 40 drops per minute
    c. 1200 units/hour
17. 1500 units/hour
18. Approximately 33 mL/hour or 33 drops per minute
19. a. Add 250 mg = 6.3 mL
    b. 5 mcg × 59 kg = 295 mcg/minute
    c. I.V. solution concentration 1 mg/mL = 1000 mcg/mL; rate of flow per minute = 0.295 mL × 60 = approximately 18 drops per minute
20. Dosage is 4 mcg × 59 kg = 236 mcg/ minute; rate of flow: approximately 14 drops per minute

Exercise 10.1

1. 3.4 mL
2. 0.92 mL
3. 0.27 mL
4. Yes; 0.34 mg is within the recommended amount
5. 2.5 mg each
6. 0.12 mL
7. 0.2 mL
8. 0.21 mL (desired dose = 1.03 kg × 50 mg = 51.5 mg)
9. Use 2 mg/mL strength; give 0.05 mL
10. Each dose is 33.13 mg; give 0.13 mL for each dose

Exercise 10.2

1. 972 mg
2. 1.87 mL
3. 37.28 mg
4. 12.57 mg
5. 0.78 sq m
6. 0.28 sq m
7. 0.58 sq m
8. 0.76 sq m

9. a. 1 500 × 0.78 sq m; 1 170 mL/day
   b. 1 500 × 0.28 sq m; 420 mL/day
   c. 1 500 × 0.58 sq m; 870 mL/day
   d. 1 500 × 0.76 sq m; 1 140 mL/day
10. a. Approximately 49 mL/hour
    b. Approximately 18 mL/hour
    c. Approximately 36 mL/hour
    d. Approximately 48 mL/hour

Exercise 10.3

1. *Problem:* dose required: 2.5 × kg
   600 g = 0.6 kg (1 000 g = 1 kg)
   Dose required = 2.5 × 0.6 = 1.5 mg
   Solution:
   Known ratio: 10 mg:1 mL
   Unknown ratio: 1.5 mg:N mL
   Proportion equation: 10 mg:1 mL = 1.5
   mg:N mL
   N = 0.15 (round to nearest hundredth = 0.15
   mL)
   Validation: 10 mg:1 mL = 1.5 mg:0.15 mL
   1 × 1.5 = 10 × 0.15
   1.5 = 1.5
Note the error that occurs with rounding;
however, most syringes are calibrated in tenths;
therefore this is acceptable.
   2a. *Problem:* calculate loading dose:
   Solution: 1 000 g:1 kg = 1 500 g:N kg
   N = 1 500 ÷ 1 000 = 1.5 kg
   Loading dose = 5 mg × 1.5 kg = 7.5mg
   Known ratio: 80 mg:15 mL
   Unknown ratio: 7.5 mg:N mL
   80:15 = 7.5:N
   80 N = 15 × 7.5
   N = 112.5 ÷ 80 = 1.406 25 (round to
   nearest hundredth: = 1.41 mL
   Validation: 80:15 = 7.5:1.406 25
   80 × 1.406 25 = 15 × 7.5
   112.5 = 112.5
   2b. Maintenance dose: 1 mg/kg ÷ 3 daily
doses
   Solution: 1 mg × 1.5 kg = 1.5 mg ÷ 3 = 0.5
   mg each dose
   Known ratio: 80 mg:15 mL
   Unknown ratio: 0.5 mg:N mL
   80:15 = 0.5:N
   80 N = 15 × 0.5 = 7.5
   N = 0.093 75 (round to nearest hundredth =
   0.09 mL)
   Validation: 80:15 = 0.5:0.093 75
   80 × 0.093 75 = 15 × 0.5
   7.5 = 7.5

3. *Problem:* dose required: 5 mcg × 0.79 kg
   = 3.95 mcg/minute at 1 mL/hour. How many
   mcg are required per hour? 3.95 mcg × 60 =
   237 mcg. How many mcg are required for 50
   mL of solution? 237 × 50 = 11 850 mcg. What
   volume of dopamine is required? Available:
   dopamine 40 mg/mL = 40 mg = 40 × 1 000
   mcg = 40 000 mcg.
   Solution: Known ratio: 40 000 mcg:mL
   Unknown ratio: 11 850 mcg:N mL
   40 000:1 = 11 850:N
   N = 0.296 25 mL; round to nearest
   hundredth = 0.30 mL
   Validation: 40 000:1 = 11 850:0.296 25
   40 000 × 0.296 25 = 11 850
   11 850 = 11 850
4. (5 mcg × 0.79 kg × 60 minutes × 50 mL)
   = 11 850 mcg dopamine in 50 mL of I.V.
solution
   11 850 mcg dopamine ÷ 40 000 mcg dopamine/
   mL = 0.296 25 mL dopamine; round to nearest
   hundredth = 0.30 mL
5. 1 mL/hour using minidrip = 1 drop per
minute
6. a. 0.5 mL/hour
   b. 0.5 drops per minute
7a. Note that formula instructions produce a
solution that delivers 5 mcg/kg/minute at 1 mL/
hour. Prepare this concentration and then run the
I.V. at 1.5 mL to deliver 7.5 mcg/kg/minute.
   5 mcg × 1.17 kg × 60 minute × 50 mL =
   17 550 mcg dopamine: 17 550 mcg dopamine ÷
   40 000 mcg dopamine = 0.438 75; round to
   nearest hundredth = 0.44 mL
Add 0.44 mL of dopamine to 50 mL of solution
and run at 1.5 mL/hour.
   7b. 526.5 mcg/hour
8. *Solution:* dose required = 3.1 × 0.03 =
   0.093 mg; round to nearest hundredth = 0.09
   mg; give 0.9 ml.
   Validation: 0.1 mg:1 mL = 0.09 mg:N mL
   0.1:1 = 0.09:0.9
   0.09 = 0.09
9. *Solution:* dose required = 1.345 kg × 1
   mg = 1.345 mg;
   round to nearest hundredth = 1.35 mg;
   Known ratio: 20 mg:mL
   Unknown ratio: 1.35 mg:N mL
   20:1 = 1.35:N
   20 N = 1.35
   N = 0.0675; round to nearest hundredth =
   0.07 mL

Validation: 20:1 = 1.35:0.0675
  20 × 0.0675 = 1.35
  1.35 = 1.35
10. 0.2 mcg × 1.265 kg × 60 = 15.18 mcg/
  hour

Exercise 10.4

1. a. 500 mg
   b. 1 mg
   c. 500 mg
   d. 10 mg
   e. 200 mg
   f. 1 mg
   g. 40 mg
   h. 1 mg
   i. 100 mg
   j. 1 g
   k. 20 mg
   l. 5 mg
   m. 500 mg
   n. 10 mg
2. 250 mg in 250 mL = 1 mg/mL
1 mg = 1 000 mcg; therefore concentration is
1 000 mcg/mL
3. $\dfrac{3.5\,\text{mcg} \times 67\,\text{kg} \times 60\,\text{minute}}{1\,000\,\text{mcg/mL}} = 14.07$
4. a. 19 drops per minute
   b. 31 drops per minute
   c. 42 drops per minute
5. a. 1 mg
   b. 30 drops per minute
   c. 3 mcg/minute × 15 minutes = 45 mcg
6. a. 8 mcg/mL
   b. 8 drops per minute
   c. 3 mcg/minute
7. 100 mg:5 mL = give 5 mL (use 20 mg/mL
strength)
8. Add 2 g to 500-mL bag; use 2 50-mL
single-dose vials of 1 g/50 mL;
infuse at 60 mL/hour (60 drops per minute)
9. For pronestyl 1 g
   100 mg:1 mL = 1 000 mg:N mL
   100 N = 1 000
   N = 10 Answer: Use 10 mL (two 5-mL
   ampules)
Validation: 100 m:1 mL = 1 000 mg:10 mL
10. Preparation: add 2 g to 500 mL of I.V.
solution
   100 mg:1 mL = 2 000 mg:N mL
   100 N = 2 000

N = 20; Answer: add 20 mL to 500-mL bag;
each ampule contains 5 mL; therefore 4
ampules are needed;
infuse at 60 drops per minute
11. 20 mg:1 mL = 100mg:N mL
   20 N = 100
   N = 5; Answer: use 1 5-mL ampule.
Validation: 20 mg:1 mL = 100 mg:5 mL
12. 5 mg/mL; give 1 mL
13. 1 mg:1 mL = 3 mg:N mL
   N = 3; Answer: give 3 mL from 5-mL
ampule.
14. Add 2 g to 500 mL
   1 g:50 mL = 2 g:N mL. Available —
   N = 100 mL; Answer: give 100 mL (use two
   50-mL ampules);
infuse at 15 drops per minute
15. 10 mg:1 mL = 20 mg:N mL
   N = 2; Answer: give 2 mL
16. Available: dopamine 40 mg/mL
Preparation of solution: add 200 mg to 500 mL
   40 mg:1 mL = 200 mg:N mL
   40 N = 200
   N = 5; Answer: add 5 mL to 500-mL bag.
Calculate rate of flow.
Find 3 mcg/minute in left-hand column and
follow line to 70 kg. Answer is 31 drops per
minute (or mL/hour).
17. *Alternative 1:* use formula
Concentration of solution: 200 mg in 500 mL =
   400 mcg/mL
   $\dfrac{4\,\text{mcg} \times 71\,\text{kg} \times 60\,\text{minutes}}{400\,\text{mcg}} = 42.6$ drops per
   minute = 43 drops per minute
Alternative 2:
Find 4 mcg/minute in left-hand column and
follow line to 70 kg. Answer is 42 drops per
minute (or mL/hour).
18. 0.1 mg:1 mL = 0.5 mg:N mL
   0.1 N = 0.5
   N = 5; Answer: give 5 mL from 10-mL
   ampule.
Validation: 0.1 mg:1 mL = 0.5 mg:5 mL
19. Add 2 mg to 500 mL of I.V. fluid = 4 mcg/
mL. Available strength: 5-mL ampule of 1 mg/5
mL.
   1 mg:5 mL = 2 mg:N mL
   N = 10; Answer: add 10 mL to 500-mL bag;
   use two 5-mL ampules;
infuse at 30 drops per minute
20. 2 mcg:minute = 30 drops:minute
   2 mcg:30 drops = 2.5 mcg:N drops
   2 N = 75

N = 37.5 or 38
Answer: increase rate to 38 drops per minute

Posttest

1. 875 mg
2. Yes; this dose is 10 mg/kg
3. No; it is lower than the recommended dosage of 1 050 daily
4. 3 tablets
5. 0.25 mL
6. 1.21 mL
7. 12.57 mg
8. 0.21 g or 213 mg
9. 650 mg
10. 0.55 mL
11. 126 mcg/minute
12. 7.2 drops per minute
13. 200 mcg/minute
14. 0.23 mL
15. 2.24 mL
16. 0.78 mL
17. 3.9 mL
18. 237 mcg/minute
19. 14 drops per minute
20. 17 drops per minute

Appendix A

1. 7.9
2. 11.9
3. 2.03
4. 69.39
5. 40.28
6. 2.62
7. 22.78
8. 8.57
9. 10.45
10. 6.85
11. 3.302
12. 0.548
13. 8.716
14. 10.992
15. 0.977
16. 136.165
17. 197.741

18. 1.968
19. 12.583
20. 23.377

Appendix B

1. 15 apples; 3:5 = 9:N
2. 15 grade three students; 8:12 = 10:N
3. Approximately 35 baskets; 18:25 = N:49
4. 1.5 cups; 1:2 = N:3
5. 20 blue beads; 5:12 = N:48
6. #1 100 mg:2 mL = 75 mg:N mL
#2 100 mg:75 mg = 2 mL:N mL
#3 2 mL:100 mg = N mL:75 mg
#4 2 mL:N mL = 100 mg:75 mg
Solution: 1.5 mL
7. #1 1 mg:10 mL = 0.4 mg:N mL
#2 1 mg:0.4 mg = 10 mL:N mL
#3 10 mL:1 mg = N mL:0.4 mg
#4 10 mL:N mL = 1 mg:0.4 mg
Solution: 4 mL
8. 200 mg = N mcg   1 mg = 1 000 mcg
1 mg:1 000 mcg = 200 mg:N mcg
N = 200 000 mcg
200 000 mcg:250 mL = N mcg:1 mL
N = 800
Answer: 800 mcg/mL
Validation: 200 000 mcg:250 mL = 800 mcg: 1
        mL
        200 000 = 200 000
9. 1 g:5 mL = N g:mL
1 g = 1 000 mg
1 000 mg:5 mL = N mg:1 mL
5 N = 1 000
N = 200
Answer: 200 mg/mL
Validation: 1 000:5 = 200:1
    1 000 = 1 000
10. 112.5 mg:5 mL = N mg:1 mL
    N = 22.5
Answer: 22.5 mg/mL
Validation: 112.5 mg:5 mL = 22.5:1 mL
    112.5 = 112.5

Appendix C

Section One

1. a. 2 tablets
   b. 4
   c. 8
2. 3 tablets
3. 2 tablets
4. 3 tablets
5. 1.5 tablet
6. 1 tablet (note 1 000 mcg = 1 mg:125 mcg = 0.125 mg)
7. 2 tablets
8. 2 tablets (0.65 g = 625 mg)
9. 2 tablets (0.05 g = 50 mg)
10. 3 tablets (1.5 g = 1 500 mg)

Section Two

1. 10 mg:1 mL = 7.5 mg:N mL
   10 N = 7.5
   N = 0.75
Answer: give 0.75 mL
Validation: 10:1 = 7.5:0.75
   Multiply the means and the extremes
   10 × 0.75 = 1 × 7.5
   7.5 = 7.5
2. 100 units:1 mL = 22 units:N mL
   100 N = 22
   N = 0.22 mL of NPH insulin
Validation: 100:1 = 22:0.22
   Multiply the means and the extremes
   100 × 0.22 = 1 × 22
   22 = 22
   100 units:1 mL = 12 units:N mL
   100 N = 12
   N = 0.12 mL of regular insulin
Validation: 100:1 = 12:0.12
   100 × 0.12 = 1 × 12
   12 = 12
Give 0.22 mL of NPH and 0.12 regular insulin
= 0.34 mL
3. 100 mg:2 mL = 75 mg:N mL
   100 N = 150

N = 1.5
Answer: give 1.5 mL
Validation: 100:2 = 75:1.5
   Multiply the means and the extremes
   100 × 1.5 = 2 × 75
   150 = 150
4. 50 mg:1 mL = 75 mg:N mL
   50 N = 75
   N = 1.5
Answer: give 1.5 mL
Validation: 50:1 = 75: 1.5
   Multiply the means and the extremes
   50 × 1.5 = 1 × 75
   75 = 75
5. 25 mg:1 mL = 12.5 mg:N mL
   25 N = 12.5
   N = 0.5
Answer: give 0.5 mL
Validation: 25:1 = 12.5:0.5
   Multiply the means and the extremes
   25 × 0.5 = 1 × 12.5
   12.5 = 12.5
6. 10 000 units:1 mL = 6 000 units:N mL
   10 000 N = 6 000
   N = 0.6
Answer: give 0.6 mL
Validation: 10 000:1 = 6 000:0.6
   Multiply the means and the extremes
   10 000 × 0.6 = 1 × 6 000
   6 000 = 6 000
7. 0.25 g = 250 mg (1 000 mg/g)
   250 mg:1.5 mL = 500 mg:N mL
   250 N = 750
   N = 3
Answer: give 3 mL
Validation: 250:1.5 = 500:3
   Multiply the means and the extremes
   250 × 3 = 1.5 × 500
   750 = 750
8. 1 oz = 30 mL
9. 1 to 2 tsp
10. 0.25 g = 250 mg (1 000 mg = 1 gram)
   250 mg:1 mL = 500 mg:N mL
   250 N = 500
   N = 2
Answer: give 2 mL
Validation: 250:1 = 500:2
   Multiply the means and the extremes
   250 × 2 = 1 × 500
   500 = 500

Section Three

1. 1% solution, 10 mg per mL
2. 50 mg
3. 1 g of drug in 100 mL of solution
(1 000 mg in 100 mL = 10 mg/mL)
4. 10 000 units/mL × 4 mL = 40 000 units
5. 10 000 units/mL
6. 5 mg
7. 5 days (25 1-mL vials)
8. 1 000 times stronger
9. 4 mL
10. 0.5 g/2.2 mL

Section Four

1. Add 4 mL diluent: concentration = 0.5 g in
2.2 mL
0.5 g = 500 mg
500 mg:2.2 mL = 250 mg:N mL
500 N = 550
N = 1.1 mL
Give 1.1 mL
Validation: 500:2.2 = 250:1.1
  Multiply the means and the extremes
  500 × 1.1 = 2.2 × 250
  550 = 550
2. Add 4 mL diluent: concentration = 0.5 g in
2.2 mL
0.5 g = 500 mg
500 mg:2.2 mL = 750 mg:N mL
500 N = 1 650
N = 3.3 mL
Give 3.3 mL
Validation: 500:2.2 = 750:3.3
  Multiply the means and the extremes
  500 × 3.3 = 2.2 × 750
  1 650 = 1 650

3. If 7 mL of diluent is added, concentration is
1 g in 2 mL. Give 2 mL.
4. 1 500 mg = 1.5 g (1 000 mg = 1 gram)
1 g:2 mL = 1.5 g:N mL
  N = 3 mL
Give 3 mL
Validation: 1:2 = 1.5:3
  Multiply the means and the extremes
  3 = 3
(Note: you may have stated the known ratio in
another way such as: 1 000 g in 2 mL or 500 mg
in 1 mL. The answer will be the same.)
5. Adding 9.5 mL diluent = 1 g/2.5 mL
17 mL diluent = 1 g/4 mL
Answer: adding 9.5 mL diluent
6. Solution concentration is 1 g/2.5 mL
1 g:2.5 mL = N g:2 mL
  2.5 N = 2
  N = 0.8
Answer: patient received 0.8 g (or 800 mg)
7. Solution concentration is 0.5 g/2.2 mL
  0.5 g:2.2 mL = N g:1 mL
  2.2 N = 0.5
  N = 0.23 g
Answer: patient received 0.23 g or 227 mg
8. At least 4 mL
9. Add 2 mL diluent: solution concentration =
1 g/2.6 mL
Give 2.6 mL.
10. Figure A.

RULES FOR ARITHMETIC OF FRACTIONS

To add fractions: find the common denominator; convert each fraction to an equivalent fraction using the common denominator; add the numerators; place the sum over the denominator; simplify

To subtract fractions: find the common denominator; convert each fraction to an equivalent fraction using the common denominator; subtract the numerators; place the sum over the denominator; simplify

To multiply fractions: multiply the numerators; multiply the denominators; place the product of the numerators over the product of the denominators; simplify

To divide fractions: invert the terms of the divisor (the number that is being divided into the dividend); use multiplication of fractions

To simplify a fraction: divide the numerator and denominator by the same number

RULES FOR ARITHMETIC OF MIXED NUMBERS

To add mixed numbers: add the whole numbers; add the fractions and simplify if necessary; combine the two sums

To subtract mixed numbers: subtract the whole numbers—or convert the mixed numbers to improper fractions; subtract the fractions and simplify if necessary

To multiply mixed numbers: express the mixed number as an improper fraction and proceed for multiplication of fractions

To divide mixed numbers: express the mixed number as an improper fraction and proceed for division of fractions